# THE COMPLETE BOOK OF ALLERGY CONTROL

Here's what they're saying about *the only book that provides a step-by-step allergy self-detection method and gives complete answers to questions concerning allergies and allergy-related illness:*

"Sound advice . . . Stevens directs readers in keeping diaries of symptoms and exposures, and explains how to analyze the two to see if allergy is indeed the problem; she also describes what medical diagnosis and treatment will entail."

—*Kirkus Reviews*

"Recommended . . . She explains how to track down specific allergens, and suggests nonallergenic substitutes. She presents detailed rotation and elimination diets for identifying food allergies, along with five chapters of recipes. The book includes a section on what to feed an infant at various ages, in order to avoid the development of allergies. Other chapters cover improving the diet and reducing stress, which can worsen allergic symptoms."

—*Library Journal*

". . . An informative book that should be particularly useful to those who have multiple or nontraditional allergies that may not be easily detected or may be misdiagnosed."

—*ALA Booklist*

# THE COMPLETE BOOK OF

# Allergy Control

LAURA J. STEVENS

Foreword by William G. Crook, M.D.

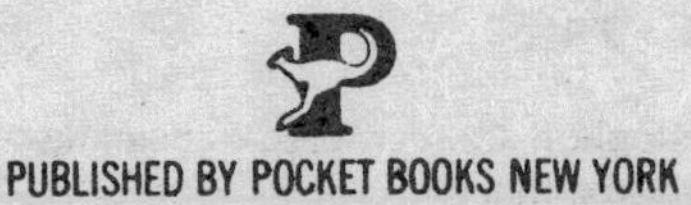

PUBLISHED BY POCKET BOOKS NEW YORK

This book is not intended as a substitute for medical advice of physicians. The reader should regularly consult a physician in matters relating to his or her health and particularly in respect of any symptoms which may require diagnosis or medical attention.

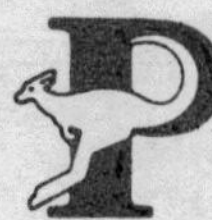

POCKET BOOKS, a division of Simon & Schuster, Inc.
1230 Avenue of the Americas, New York, N.Y. 10020



Published by arrangement with Macmillan Publishing Company
Library of Congress Catalog Card Number: 83-12085



ISBN: 0-671-50886-5

First Pocket Books printing March, 1986

10 9 8 7 6 5 4 3 2 1



Printed in the U.S.A.

*For George, Jack, Jeff, David,*
*Mary, Lana, Helen,*
*Diane, Cheryl, Margie, and . . .*

# FOREWORD

At a time when most physicians and professional medical organizations are urging the layman to learn more about how to be well and stay well rather than to rely on the medical profession for "a quick fix" or a "magic pill" for every ache or pain, Laura Stevens's well-researched and documented book is a welcome addition to the shelf of responsible self-help medical books.

The identification, definition, and treatment of allergies and allergy-related illness is often frustrating and confusing because allergists, like members of opposing political parties, subscribe to very different views. The traditional allergists rather strictly define the causes and effects of allergies, while the nontraditional allergists acknowledge a much broader range of allergens and reactions to them.

Like everyone else, I knew that allergies could make people sneeze, wheeze, and itch but I didn't know that nervousness, muscle aches, hyperactivity, arthritis, and depression could be caused by sensitivity to inhalants, foods, and chemicals. And, although my chief during my pediatric internship and residency at Vanderbilt University Hospital had told me that I would see more allergy-related symptoms and illness in my practice than I expected, I had only a smattering of knowledge of allergies and little interest in the subject at the end of my medical training.

Once in private practice a few years later, an alert mother convinced me (somewhat against my will) that her twelve-year-old's headaches, irritability, fatigue, and nervousness vanished when milk was eliminated from his diet. Soon after, I read an article by Dr. Frederick Speer of the University of Kansas in *The Pediatric Clinics of North America* that reported a marked improvement in the behavior of children whose diets excluded foods such as milk, eggs, corn, and wheat, and I then began my own studies of the effect of certain foods on children's behavior, which was published in *Pediatrics* in 1961. At the same time, I was learning that sensitivity to certain foods made many of my adult patients pale, tired, and nervous.

During the sixties and seventies my interest in food allergies and nutrition grew as I became familiar with the work of Roger J. Williams, Ph.D., Emmanual Cheraskin, M.D., D.M.D., and Linus Pauling, Ph.D., while continually observing the relationship among my own patients between certain symptoms and disorders and what they ate. I was excited to find that many of their physical and psychological symptoms could be alleviated simply by a change in diet.

The work of pioneer allergist and clinical ecologist, Theron Randolph, M.D., alerted me to the fact that food additives, air pollutants, odorous plastics, perfumes, tobacco, and other environmental chemicals made many of my patients sick; and Birmingham allergist Orian Truss, M.D., introduced me to Candida albicans, a yeast that weakens the body's immune system while causing chronic illness and aggravation of allergies.

The rather narrow field of allergy that I had at first found uninteresting has emerged as one of the most vital, important, and controversial areas in modern medicine.

*The Complete Book of Allergy Control* provides a clear and comprehensive analysis of the traditional and nontraditional views of allergy and a concise overview of the relationship of allergy to a wide variety of health problems. Procedures for allergy detection, treatment, prevention, and control are clear and effective, and the chapters on nutrition and vitamin and mineral supplements clarify the many confusing issues related to nutrition and health. Environmental pollutants and their effects and what can be done to lessen exposure to them is a particularly important and useful section of the book. Also included is valuable information about RAST and cytoxic tests and the more controversial methods of provocative testing and of neutralizing reactions to foods and chemicals as well as a succinct summary of the very recent "medical breakthroughs" linking the yeast Candida albicans and the mercury in dental fillings to increased susceptibility to allergic symptoms.

Laura Stevens wrote this book to help those afflicted with chronic, undiagnosed symptoms understand the complex subject of allergy-related illness, and she has done this better and more thoroughly than any other writer covering the territory. But the book's usefulness does not end with the layman. *The Complete Book of Allergy Control* should be in the hands of every physician whose patients' complaints may be caused by allergy, the environment, or nutrition—and in my opinion that includes almost everybody.

*Jackson, Tennessee, 1983*

—WILLIAM G. CROOK, M.D.
Fellow of The American Academy of Pediatrics, The American College of Allergists, and The Society for Clinical Ecology

# ACKNOWLEDGMENTS

Many people have helped make this book possible, but I'd like especially to thank the following: my family, for their encouragement and patience; John F. O'Brian, M.D., who has helped our family through thick and thin, and his nurses, Dorothy Boyce, R.N., and Evelyn Buck, for their tender loving care and continuing courses in allergy education; William Crook, M.D., for his advice, support, and suggestions over the years; Lendon Smith, M.D., for steering us toward nutritional therapies; C. Orian Truss, M.D., for helping us with his comprehensive anti-yeast program and giving us hope that we would get well; Donald Rudin, M.D., for his guidance in using essential fatty acids; Hal Huggins, D.D.S., and Richard Ellsworth, D.D.S., for opening my eyes to the dangers of mercury in silver fillings and the importance of balancing body chemistry.

Thanks also go to Mary Wachs, Ph.D., for her demonstration of relaxation therapy; to Kathryn Black, Ph.D., for her enlightening view of the psychological problems of being allergic; and to James Ascough, Ph.D., for his help with biofeedback and relaxation. Finally, thanks to all the members of our Allergy Awareness Group, who have become my good friends and taught me many new things about allergy.

# INTRODUCTION

Do you have allergies? You may not think you do. Your doctor may never have mentioned it. But you still may have them. Even if your nose doesn't run, you never wheeze, and your skin doesn't break out in a rash, you may have other symptoms. And they may be caused by allergies. Are you, for instance, always tired even though you get enough sleep? Do you have headaches, joint pains, or intestinal upsets? Are you feeling depressed? Confused? Do you have difficulty concentrating?

You may already have gone from doctor to doctor in a frustrating search for the cause of your symptoms. And the doctors may be puzzled. What disease could possibly cause such a variety of symptoms? None of the tests shows anything. Assuring you that nothing's wrong doesn't help much. You still feel lousy. You know you're not a hypochondriac. But what can you do?

Many doctors are beginning to recognize that allergies can cause all kinds of symptoms—headaches, a sore knee, insomnia, stomach cramps, and many others. The severity can range from occasional, mild attacks to crippling mental and physical problems. Identifying the offending substances can dramatically change the person's life. For many, the solution may be as easy as finding out that chocolate brings on headaches. For others, the answers may be more complex. But as one doctor remarked, "What is not looked for will never be found!" If you never search for your allergies, you'll never find any.

Your symptoms may not be nearly as severe as those of my family, but perhaps our experiences will introduce you to a new, broader view of allergies. All of us suffered from unexplained illnesses. Sometimes allergies were the major cause; other times, it was more that allergies were a contributing factor, making us feel worse. And the underlying culprits in our allergies may well have promoted other illnesses.

I've had allergies almost all my life. My older brother had asthma and hay fever almost from day one. Before I was born, the doctor warned my parents that I might be allergic too, since allergies often run in families. Surprisingly, as a baby, I didn't have any allergies. But by the time I was a toddler, my first allergy appeared—chocolate ice cream made my nose stream. Unfortunately, many other foods began to make my nose run. Eliminating them from my diet seemed to keep my nose clear. It really wasn't a big sacrifice—my brother and mother had food allergies, too. But I did miss chocolate ice cream and cake at birthday parties.

Several years later my nost started streaming every spring with the grass pollens. A simple antihistamine kept it under control. Then, I began to react to the animals at the zoo and had to miss out on our school's Zoo Day. Exhaust fumes made me carsick. Wet paint gave me headaches. Sulfa made my face break out in welts. I always developed a severe local infection after a bee sting. Still, by and large, I was healthy and happy. My allergies seemed just a minor annoyance.

When I was a senior in high school, however, I came down with a severe case of "flu." I dragged to school for several weeks before giving in to the throbbing headaches, leg pains, fatigue, and depression. My doctor diagnosed the flu as a viral brain infection (encephalitis), which was later confirmed at the Mayo Clinic. All the doctors assured me I would get better. But to a seventeen-year-old with college plans, recovery seemed to take forever. In fact, I was in bed for about a year and a half. The headaches seemed intolerable; the leg pains wouldn't go away. At first I slept and slept, but no matter how much I slept, I always felt exhausted. I became very depressed because I felt so crummy. All kinds of pills were tried, but nothing really worked. In fact, they made things worse, for I had adverse reactions to most of the drugs. Years later, I still wonder where the virus stopped and my adult allergies began. Certainly I was very ill during those years. There was no doubt I had encephalitis. But in coming to understand my allergies, I have begun to wonder if the viral disease might not have been compounded by allergies. Treating allergies alone isn't the answer—but one shouldn't ignore them either.

In any case, my appetite was poor and my diet was a disaster. I'd lost so much weight that my parents and doctor were delighted when I was interested in any kind of food. Yet at a time when my body needed nutritious food to recover, I fed it mostly junk. Soft drinks tasted good, slipped down easily, and seemed to perk me up. I began to drink them more and more. Soon I was hooked—a "cola-holic." I had other strong food cravings, but not for anything particularly nourishing.

On top of it all, I had increasingly severe menstrual pains every month—almost incapacitating. Doctor after doctor prescribed birth control pills, but each kind made me vomit. Years later I learned that birth control pills severely aggravate chronic yeast infections, one of the newly recognized factors that may promote allergies (see Chapter 9). Nor did the birth control pills help my menstrual pains. Finally, one doctor diagnosed my problem as endometriosis. Surgery alleviated the pain—for a few months. (It's only recently that I've learned how often women with chronic yeast infections suffer from endometriosis and other menstrual disorders—perhaps due to the hormonal imbalance.)

At long last I started college. My illness had changed my career plans; I majored in biology with the hope of going to medical school. But my health was still a problem. I was always exhausted and seemed to pick up every infection that went around. The worst was the year I took organic chemistry and an anatomy class. I remember having to dissect a dead cat preserved in formaldehyde. I took that cat everywhere; I even kept it in my bedroom at night. It puzzled and frustrated me. Everyone else seemed to learn the cat's anatomy easily, but I couldn't remember the name of a muscle from one day to the next. And it wasn't only that I couldn't concentrate. I also developed pain and stiffness in my hands and knees—not to mention depression. What a year! Since then, I've learned how sensitive I am to chemicals, especially formaldehyde.

Although my grades were good, medical school was out of the question. So I changed my major and went to graduate school in political science. There I met my future husband, George. (Sometimes things work out for the best after all!) But however happy I was, life was not all rosy. My severe menstrual problems continued. Again, surgery was unsuccessful. The surgeon urged George and me to start a family as soon as possible because I might have trouble becoming pregnant. If the pain continued after I had children, then a hysterectomy could be performed.

So George and I got married and moved to Indiana. I started a job in a nearby university's horticulture department, working with plants and chemicals galore. Little did I realize at the time how much the moldy greenhouse and the chemicals were aggravating my fatigue and achiness.

Soon I became pregnant. Everything was okay until the fifth month, when premature labor started for no apparent reason. For the next few months, I was in and out of the hospital, holding off birth. Finally, Jack was born safe and sound, three weeks early.

We didn't know much about raising children, but we were excited about Jack—a beautiful, lively baby. Soon, however, Jack was screaming with colic, and this continued for nine long months. We changed formulas, but he screamed as much on soy as on cow's milk. We started solids early; he seemed hungry and the doctor said to try them. Nothing helped. Jack was hospitalized at four months and again at eight months. But no physical cause for the colic could be found. The doctor eventually concluded that tension was the cause.

Yes, we were tense! George had had his gallbladder out the month before Jack was born. Three months after Jack's birth, I started having gallbladder attacks that wouldn't stop. So, I, too, had gallbladder surgery. Then, when Jack was six months old, I came down with a severe viral infection. The doctor suspected I had another form of encephalitis. What luck!

Somehow Jack's colic subsided, but our problems were not over. Yes, at times Jack seemed happy, but it was a case of Dr. Jekyll-Mr. Hyde. One moment he was sweet, and lovable; the next he was irritable and screaming. Jack seemed especially sensitive to loud noises. He was always bouncing or rocking and quickly wore out two crib mattresses. Frequent temper tantrums plagued his toddler years. We read through all the psychology books we could find, but they never seemed to describe Jack's problems.

During this time my own health was up and down. I had bouts of joint pain and stiffness. My "gallbladder" attacks continued for a year, even though I had no gallbladder. I was forever getting bladder infections—and every other kind of infection. I ran a low-grade fever. No matter how much I slept, I was tired. No one could pinpoint what was wrong.

After consulting several psychologists, we finally took Jack to see a pediatric neurologist, who diagnosed Jack as severely hyperactive. He put Jack on Ritalin, a drug used to calm hyperactive children. By then I had read about allergist Ben Feingold's diet for hyperactive children. The diet eliminates artificial food colorings and flavorings, as well as natural foods that contain an aspirinlike chemical. I asked the doctor whether there was anything to this diet. In his opinion, it was just a fad.

But the Ritalin didn't work. What were we to do? In desperation, we tried Dr. Feingold's diet. Within five days, Jack had dramatically improved. He was calm, reasonable, and seemed happy all the time. His speech was clearer; he played better with other children; his attention span increased. Obviously he felt good about himself.

In the midst of all this our second son, Jeff, was born—right before Jack was three. Again, I had premature labor—this time, within two weeks of Jeff's conception. I spent the next eight months in and out of the hospital on narcotics and intravenous alcohol, trying to keep him from being born prematurely. He was six weeks early but arrived safe and sound—another beautiful son.

Jeff, too, had colic, but his lasted only three months. At ten weeks, however, he had severe projectile vomiting. Surgery for suspected pyloric stenosis, a defect in the passageway from the stomach to the intestines, was performed. After surgery, the defect was found to be less severe than expected, and the surgeon then concluded that food allergy was the major cause of the vomiting. Although Jeff continued to have trouble keeping his formula down, on the whole he was a very placid baby. In fact, he seemed too placid; it worried me. But the doctor assured me he was fine. He was just so different from Jack.

Several months after Jeff was born, I finally had the hysterectomy. My health did improve. It was a relief not to have all that abdominal pain. But I was still exhausted, with various aches and pains on and off. Maybe it was just "battle fatigue" from the various problems with the children. And those problems never seemed to stop.

At eighteen months, Jeff had no speech whatsoever. We had him tested. His hearing was fine, but the specialist told us to have his speech checked every six months. Jeff still hadn't said anything by age two and very little by age two and a half. He started speech therapy. Then, our placid baby began to have "night terrors." He would awake screaming and run around the house, out of control. And the night terrors became day terrors, with the same behavior. We were exhausted, worried, and confused. What could cause such diverse problems? Only later did we learn that Jeff's slow speech was allergy-related, and his bizarre behavior stemmed from multiple food allergies.

Jack who had started kindergarten, was still on the Feingold diet. I began to notice that he reacted to many natural foods, too—soy, egg, chicken, wheat, rye, oats, and rice. The list grew. Not knowing what to make of this, I began to read what other doctors besides Dr. Feingold were writing. William Crook's excellent *Can*

*Your Child Read? Is He Hyperactive?* was a real eye-opener. Maybe we were dealing with allergies! Not your typical allergies, like the runny noses my brother and I had as children, but behavioral reactions to foods and other substances.

Then I read pediatrician Lendon Smith's *Improving Your Child's Behavior Chemistry* and *Feed Your Kids Right*. Dr. Smith writes compellingly of the need for good nutrition for every child. He urges parents to take problem children off milk, and all children off sugar and refined flour. He also recommends specific vitamins and minerals to calm the difficult child and to help the body fight off allergies and disease. Following his advice certainly seemed to help.

We found an excellent doctor some miles from us who offered special allergy testing and treatment for hyperactive and learning-disabled children. During testing we witnessed again all the symptoms Jack had had earlier, when he'd eaten the offending foods—irritability, aching legs, bloating, runny nose, short attention span, rocking back and forth.

And I soon learned that food reactions were not limited to the hyperactive child. One night we were all eating plain popcorn. Jeff, who had been sitting quietly, suddenly looked bloated, then started tearing around the house. He was allergic to corn! Special allergy testing confirmed just how sensitive he was to corn and many other foods.

As I listened to the stories of our doctor's other allergy patients, I soon realized that my fatigue, aching joints, depression, even my addiction to soft drinks, were all symptoms of my allergies. No, my nose didn't stream anymore, but I was still allergic. The symptoms had just changed form.

Food wasn't the only culprit. I read Theron Randolph's books—*Human Ecology and Susceptibility to the Chemical Environment* and, later, *An Alternative Approach to Allergies* (written with Ralph Moss). For over thirty years, Dr. Randolph has worked with children and adults whose sensitivities to inhalants and chemicals caused a wide variety of physical and emotional problems. Firsthand I observed through special allergy testing how exposure to molds, dust, pollens, and chemicals would cause my sons to be hyperactive and irritable, and how I became tired, achy, and depressed. My curiosity was aroused, and I began reading everything I could find on allergies and nutrition (see the suggested reading in Appendix F).

Our allergies are well under control now. An exciting new treatment for chronic yeast infection is helping our immune systems recover from our multiple allergies, with full recovery the objective. Both children are doing well in school and are a joy to have around—as long as we stick to our diets and allergy treatments. Physically, I have lots more energy; my joints and muscles rarely ache; and I don't get every bug that makes the rounds. Mentally, I don't get depressed; I'm alert and cope well with the ups and downs of normal life. I feel good about myself and can enjoy life. My husband, too, has found he has allergies. He knows that wheat makes him feel hungry, corn and milk make him puffy and upset his hiatal hernia. Artificial colorings turn him into an insomniac. Probably if we had a dog or cat, it would have allergies too! Our problems may be severe, but we're not that unusual. Lots of people have allergies; they're just not *aware* of them.

*Awareness* is the key. Once you are aware that coffee aggravates your arthritis, that fluorescent lighting makes you irritable and tired, that the formaldehyde in particle board and insulation gives you severe headaches, or that molds bring on depression and aching muscles, you can modify your environment to minimize exposure to the offending substances. People have always had to adapt to their environments in one way or another to survive. This is no less true today.

The purpose of this book is to make you more aware of what your environment may be doing to your health, how you can identify offending substances, and what you can do to cope with these problems. Obviously, if you haven't been feeling well, the *first* step is to see your doctor for a complete physical. But if your symptoms remain unexplained, allergy might be the hidden cause. Caution is needed, however. *If your symptoms are chronic or severe, don't attempt self-treatment.* Consult a doctor who is interested in and knowledgeable about treating problems with a nutritional or allergic origin.

Now it's time to begin your search for allergies. Good luck!

# SECTION ONE

# What Is an Allergy?

# 1

# The Traditional View of Allergies

Some 35 million Americans suffer from traditionally recognized allergy symptoms.[1] You yourself probably know many people who are allergic to one thing or another. And just think of the large number of over-the-counter remedies for allergies sold at your drugstore. Obviously, allergies are very common. Why, then, is there so much controversy among doctors about allergies?

The problem begins with the definition: What is an allergy? The term *allergy* was first coined in 1906 by an Austrian pediatrician, Clemens von Pirquet, to mean an "altered reactivity"—a reaction a person has to some specific substance that is normally harmless to other people. The offending substance is called an *allergen.*

Allergies occur when something goes wrong in the functioning of the immune system. Our white blood cells defend us from foreign substances *(antigens)* by producing certain proteins in the blood, known as *antibodies*, or immunoglobulins. Normally, this measure is taken only with harmful invaders, such as bacteria or viruses. The antibodies may combine with the foreign substances to neutralize their harmful effects, or they may eliminate them in other ways. In the allergic person, however, the immune system produces antibodies against *harmless* substances such as pollens, dust, molds, and foods. The antibodies then interact with mast cells located in the skin, the lining of the respiratory and intestinal tracts, and around tiny veins. When allergens arrive by way of the bloodstream, they combine with the antibodies, causing the mast cells to release histamine and other potent chemicals, creating inflammation, swelling, and smooth muscle contractions—an allergic reaction.

In the beginning of this century, the term *allergy* was used quite broadly to refer to an abnormal reaction to any substance. By the 1920s, however, under the influence of European allergists, the term was often restricted to reactions in which a definite antibody-antigen response would be demonstrated. The problem is that not all types of observed reactions can be explained by this antibody-antigen response. So two schools of allergists have developed—a traditional and a nontraditional one. Although these doctors agree on many facets of allergy, there are significant differences of opinion.

## ■ A NARROW VIEW OF SYMPTOMS

Traditional allergists limit the term *allergy* to reactions in which the antibody-antigen response can be demonstrated by currently available immunological or laboratory methods. Specifically, they recognize the following syndromes as frequently (although not always) caused by allergic reactions:

### Allergic Rhinitis and Hay Fever

A stuffy, running, or itchy nose; sneezing; red, watery eyes; an irritated throat—these are common symptoms of allergic rhinitis. If you have frequent "colds" that persist past a few days, you may actually be suffering from allergic rhinitis. Irritation may extend into the sinuses or down into the bronchial tubes. The tissues lining the nose tend to be pale if allergies are present, dark red if an infection is the cause. Sometimes a child's nose itches so much that the child starts rubbing with the back of the hand and continues all the way up the arm, in an "allergic salute"!

Symptoms may be seasonal or occur year-round, depending on the cause. House dust, molds, and animal danders are common offenders. Recently chemicals in the workplace have been recognized as triggers for allergic rhinitis. Treatment may involve avoidance of offending allergens, use of appropriate drugs, and desensitizing injections.

Hay fever is simply allergic rhinitis that is caused by a sensitivity to seasonal pollens such as ragweed. About 14.7 million Americans are afflicted by it.[2] But don't be misled by the name *hay fever*—it's not always caused by hay and there's no fever.

### Asthma

Some nine million Americans suffer from asthma, and acute attacks (not always triggered by allergies) kill some six thousand Americans each year.[3] Difficulty in breathing, wheezing, coughing, and a feeling of tightness in the chest characterize asthma. There are bronchial spasms, as well as heavy mucus in the bronchial tubes. House dust, molds, pollen, animal danders, and foods may provoke an asthmatic attack. Other traditionally recognized triggers include aspirin, yellow food dyes, and industrial chemicals, although in these cases the reaction is referred to as an "intolerance." Treatment consists of avoidance of known irritants and precipitating factors (such as cold air), stress reduction, breathing exercises, drug therapy, and desensitizing injections.

### Contact Dermatitis

This skin rash is characterized by redness, swelling, itching, scaliness, and blistering. It is caused by direct contact with some substance to which the skin is sensitive. Initially the rash is confined to the area where contact took place, but in severe cases the rash may spread over large areas of the body. A poison ivy or poison oak rash is the most common example. Other possible triggers include nickel, chromates, environmental and industrial chemicals, drugs, and cosmetics. A first step in treatment is to identify and remove the suspected cause. For relief of discomfort, bland topical creams, cortisone creams, or anti-itching agents may be recommended. Oral cortisone is used for severe reactions.

### Eczema

Another skin reaction—affecting nine out of every 1,000 Americans—is eczema.[4] Eczema tends to run in families; often it begins in infancy. A red, blistery, oozing rash appears on the cheeks or inner sides of the arms, legs, and wrists. This rash may simply disappear as the baby grows older, or it may persist, taking hold especially in the creases of the elbows, behind the knees, and on the fronts of the legs. With age, the rash becomes drier in nature, but other complications may arise—for instance, children with eczema frequently develop allergic rhinitis or asthma. Of course aggravating factors, such as dust, pollens, animal danders, fabrics, environmental allergens, and offending foods, need to be avoided. Antihistamines may be used to reduce the itching, along with topical cortisone creams and measures to prevent scratching and avoid infection.

**Hives (Urticaria)**

One-fifth of the U.S. population is thought to have had hives at one time or another.[5] Characterized by itchy, raised wheals or welts, this rash may appear suddenly and disappear quickly, or it may last for days. Often the offending substance is some specific food or drug, but hives may also be a reaction to pollens, insect bites, or even physical conditions such as temperature or light. Treatment consists of avoiding specific precipitating agents; antihistamines and other drugs may be used to relieve discomfort.

**Anaphylaxis**

With this serious generalized allergic reaction, there may be sudden swelling of the mucous membranes in the respiratory tract, difficulty in breathing, abdominal cramps, hives, and a drop in blood pressure, leading to collapse or even death. The cause is usually acute sensitivity to insect stings (by bees, wasps, yellow jackets, or hornets), a drug such as penicillin, or sometimes certain foods. This reaction demands emergency medical treatment, followed by measures to prevent future reactions.

## A RESTRICTED LIST OF ALLERGENS

Traditional allergists also take a narrow view of the substances that can provoke allergic symptoms, limiting those included in each category:

**Inhalants**

The term *inhalants* refers to natural airborne particles—that is, to things you breathe in. Usually you can't see these particles, but they are there suspended in the air all around you—molds, dust, pollens, and animal danders. Other common inhalant allergens include such natural particles as orrisroot (which used to be widely used in cosmetics), pyrethrum (a chemical derived from plants related to ragweed and used in insecticides), cottonseed and flaxseed (found in animal feeds, fertilizers, inexpensive upholstery, hair products, and some foods), and vegetable gums (present in some denture adhesive powders, toothpowders, hair care products, cosmetics, and many foods).[6] Traditionally recognized reactions to inhalant allergens include asthma, allergic rhinitis, and sometimes eczema and hives. Traditional testing and treatment for inhalant allergies are reliable and effective for many people.

### Foods

Foods have long been recognized as a cause of allergic reactions, although inhalant allergies are more readily accepted by doctors because the antigen-antibody response is better understood. Unfortunately, traditional allergy testing has proved unreliable with foods. What is recognized is the obvious—the person who goes into shock while eating nuts, someone who breaks out in hives after consuming strawberries, or the person who invariably vomits after drinking a glass of milk. Less clear-cut reactions tend to be overlooked. Traditional allergists remain skeptical about the connection between food allergy and neurological problems, such as behavioral disturbances or depression. They do not believe the evidence is conclusive. In addition, many traditional allergists view food allergies as mostly affecting children under the age of three, with only rare occurrences in adults.

### Other Factors

Occasionally *stinging insects* cause severe systemic allergic reactions, although this accounts for fewer than 100 deaths each year in the United States.[7] Symptoms range from hives, itching, and flushing to swelling of the voice box, severe spasms of the bronchial tubes, shock, and death. For people who have previously experienced severe reactions to insect stings, emergency self-treatment kits are available by prescription; these contain a premeasured dose of epinephrine for immediate injection. Desensitization shots are usually effective against future stings.

*Drugs*—antibiotics, aspirin, insulin, local anesthetics, and vaccines—are another common cause of allergic reactions. But not every adverse reaction to a drug is an allergy. Skin rashes, such as hives and eczema, are the most common form of drug allergy. Other allergic reactions include drug fever, anaphylaxis, asthma, other respiratory problems, and liver and kidney changes. Penicillin is the most common drug causing anaphylaxis.

Finally, traditional allergists recognize that *chemicals* and *metals* found in the workplace, cosmetics, jewelry, and foods may cause allergic rhinitis, contact dermatitis, hives, and asthma.

# 2

# The Nontraditional View of Allergies

Nontraditional allergists use the term *allergy* as it was originally defined by von Pirquet—to refer to a sensitivity, intolerance, or susceptibility to substances that don't bother the average person. Included are both reactions in which the immunological mechanisms are understood and those in which they are not. As the nontraditional allergists point out, there has always been a lag in medicine from the time when some treatment is observed to work, to when why it works is explained, to when it is accepted by the entire medical community. In the mid-nineteenth century, for instance, Ignaz Semmelweis, a Hungarian physician in Vienna, found that if he washed his hands before delivering babies, the mothers usually did not die of childbirth fever. Few doctors at the time took him seriously; in fact, he was ridiculed for his beliefs. Only some years later did Louis Pasteur discover that germs cause disease. Even more time elapsed before such cleanliness became widely accepted. Similarly, in the 1750s, the English naval surgeon James Lind observed that sailors who ate limes didn't come down with scurvy. Years passed before the discovery was made that limes contain vitamin C and that scurvy is a vitamin C-deficiency disease.

Let's look specifically at the medical controversy over the term *allergy*. What if a child has asthma attacks when exposed to molds and pollens? Doctors agree that this is an allergy. But what if the child also has asthma attacks every time certain foods are eaten or particular chemicals are present? Some doctors deny that such reactions occur. Others wouldn't want to call the reaction an allergy. What if this asthmatic child also becomes hyperactive and experiences joint pain when exposed to molds, foods, and chemicals? Is the asthma an allergy but the hyperactivity and joint pain something else? And what if another child just becomes hyperactive (without asthma) after eating foods with artificial colorings? What should this be called? Some doctors say this reaction is imagined, impossible, or very rare. Others refer to it as an "intolerance," "sensitivity," or "chemical susceptibility." Yet others do not hesitate to call this kind of reaction an "allergy." All this leaves the patient very confused!

## ■ AN EXPANDED VIEW OF SYMPTOMS

Nontraditional allergists concur that hay fever, asthma, skin rashes, and anaphylaxis are commonly caused by allergies. But they believe that these reactions represent just the tip of the "allergic iceberg," and that many less obvious symptoms are also caused by allergies, although their origin goes unsuspected. In their opinion, the respiratory system and the skin are not the only common sites of allergic reactions; any organ in the body, from the brain to the stomach to the joints, can be the target of an allergic reaction, depending on the individual.[1]

Here is a partial list of symptoms that may be due to allergies. Certainly these symptoms may have other physical or psychological causes, and these need to be *very carefully investigated by your physician.* But allergy should never be overlooked.

**Physical Symptoms**

1. *In infants:* Colic, formula intolerance, frequent spitting up, severe vomiting.
2. *General:* Low-grade fever, underweight, overweight, loss of appetite, excessive hunger.
3. *Gastrointestinal:* Canker sores, dry mouth, toothache, indigestion, heartburn, gas, nausea, vomiting, stomach ulcer, colitis, abdominal pain, gallbladder attacks, constipation, diarrhea, ileitis, hemorrhoids.
4. *Respiratory:* Coughing, mouth breathing, wheezing, asthma.
5. *Ear, Nose, Throat:* Frequent colds, runny or itchy nose, sore or tickling throat, coughing, sneezing, hay fever, nosebleeds, sinusitis, postnasal drip, nasal polyps, tonsilitis, ringing in ears, partial deafness, ear infections, dizziness.
6. *Eyes:* Puffiness, dark circles, itchiness, tearing, blurred or double vision.
7. *Skin:* Pale complexion, sweating, flushing, itching, hives, rash, pimples.
8. *Nervous system:* Headaches, migraines, dizziness, convulsions, epileptic seizures (*see also* Behavioral and Mental Symptoms).
9. *Musculoskeletal:* Weakness, leg aches, muscle pains, backaches, soreness, joint swelling or stiffness, spasms, arthritis.
10. *Cardiovascular:* Low or high blood pressure, chilling, hot flashes, faintness, heartbeat irregularities, chest pain, angina.
11. *Urinary:* Bladder infections, bed wetting, frequent painful or difficult urination, water retention.
12. *Possibly related diseases:* Low blood sugar (hypo-

glycemia), high blood sugar (diabetes), lupus, Crohn's disease, multiple sclerosis.

**Behavioral and Mental Symptoms**

1. *Irritability:* Whining, fussiness, short fuse, crying over anything.
2. *Hyperactivity:* Can't sit still, short attention span, talks too much, impulsive or compulsive behavior.
3. *Hypoactivity:* Fatigue, listlessness, drowsiness, weakness, sluggishness, sleeps too much, always tired.
4. *Clumsiness:* Accident-proneness, lack of coordination.
5. *Sleep difficulties:* Insomnia, up and down all night, nightmares, sleep apnea.
6. *Hypersensitivity:* Extreme responsiveness to odors, noise, hot/cold, light, touch; ticklishness.
7. *"Psychological" problems:* Mood swings (Dr. Jekyll-Mr. Hyde), mania, depression, confusion, spaciness, difficulty concentrating, feeling of unreality, hallucinations, anxiety, paranoia, phobias, schizophrenia.
8. *Specific Learning Problems:* Dyslexia, poor memory, poor concentration.
9. *Addictions:* Alcoholism, drug abuse, compulsive eating.

## A BROAD LOOK AT ALLERGENS

Nontraditional allergists agree with traditional allergists on the inhalants, foods, and drugs that are common allergens. But they also cite many other chemicals in our air, water, and food as causing severe psychological and physical symptoms. Some people seem to be sensitive to only one or two kinds of allergens and are not bothered by other substances—or they may not be *aware* that they have other problems. Others seem to be sensitive to just about everything (yours truly!). These super-sensitive people are "universally allergic" and have a difficult job learning what substances they can tolerate in small amounts and what substances they must totally avoid. But how do nontraditional allergists view allergy-causing substances?

**Inhalants**

Nontraditional allergists believe that molds, dust, pollens, and animal danders can cause a multitude of other symptoms in addition to traditionally recognized hay fever or asthma symptoms. These minute airborne particles enter the body through the respiratory system and are absorbed by the mucous membranes of the nose, mouth, and lungs. But that is not the end. From there on, they may affect any organ in the body. Thus, no matter what the symptoms are, nontraditional allergists carefully question their patients to see if there is a seasonal aspect to the symptoms, or if there are any other clues suggesting inhalant sensitivity (see Chapter 4).

**Foods**

Food allergy has always been controversial because its mechanism is poorly understood. Some nontraditional allergists believe that food intolerance is responsible for as much as 60% of all human illness![2] You probably know someone with a food allergy. But if food allergy is so common, why do patients and their doctors miss the connection between the foods they eat and their symptoms?

Food allergies are subtle. If you get violently sick every time you eat a food, you will quickly identify the offending food and make efforts to avoid it. But it's not always that simple. You may actually get hooked on the very substances that are making you ill. What happens is that you may feel better just after you eat the offending food. Within a few hours, however, your symptoms start to return. Given the first, immediate relief, you think that if you eat that food again you'll feel better. So you eat more. That's *food addiction!* Sometimes sensitive people live like this for years, more or less keeping their symptoms in check. This kind of food allergy is called *masked, hidden,* or *delayed-onset food allergy.*

So your cravings for certain foods may indicate that you're sensitive to them; they may be an important clue in uncovering the causes of unexplained symptoms. Any other foods eaten frequently are also suspect. But here's some better news: Foods that you despise are often culprits. You know instinctively that eating that food doesn't make you feel good. Yet you may be eating that food in other forms. For instance, you may hate eating eggs, but eggs are an ingredient in many other common foods, such as baked goods.

Another important point to remember is that the symptoms of your allergy may change with age. Let's say you're allergic to milk. As a baby, you may be colicky; as a four-year-old, you may suffer from frequent ear infections; as a teenager, you may have headaches, and perhaps arthritis as an adult. The cause of these symptoms remains the same (cow's milk); only the symptoms have changed. (By the way, milk allergy is the only specific food allergy that seems to run in families. Frequently, if a child is milk-sensitive so is someone else in the family—one or both parents, siblings, other relatives.)

Here is another confusing aspect of food allergies: The relation between symptoms and offending foods varies enormously from person to person, and even in the same person. Some people have just one symptom, but it is caused by many different foods. You may, for example, develop a headache every time you eat wheat, corn, milk, and chocolate. *Or* you may show several different symptoms with the same food. You may experience depression, nausea, and aching joints every time you eat eggs. *Or* you may have different symptoms with different foods. You may become depressed on sugar, get a headache from wheat, have a runny nose with eggs, and itch on pork! *Or,* finally, you may experience different symptoms at different times from the same food. One day drinking milk may bring on fatigue, another day milk may cause aching muscles, and on yet another occasion, a streaming nose. All this is very confusing if you're not aware of the variabilities of food allergy.

Except for *pure* salt or water, *any* food substance can bother you. The most likely culprits are the foods you eat most frequently. For most Americans, these are:

—Cow's milk (includes ice cream, butter, yogurt, cheese).
—Eggs.
—Sugar (both cane and beet).
—Citrus fruits.
—Chocolate, cola drinks, coffee.
—Corn (includes corn syrup, corn starch, corn-distilled liquor).
—Wheat, rye, barley (includes grain-distilled liquor).

Other foods commonly causing reactions are certain vegetables and fruits (tomatoes, potatoes, onions, peas, berries, apples), some meats (beef, pork), chicken, fish, peanuts, soy, certain spices (cinnamon), cottonseed, and yeast (baker's and brewer's).

Most food allergies are *unfixed*—meaning that if you

eliminate an offending food for a certain length of time (usually one to two months) and then reintroduce it on a rotation basis (once every four or five days), you will be able to tolerate that food. A *fixed* food allergy always produces symptoms; the offending food cannot be reintroduced.

*The Special Dangers of Sugar.* One food to be particularly wary of is sugar. Everyone needs to eat sugar for energy, right? Wrong, say nontraditional allergists. They have observed that sugar often causes or aggravates a variety of symptoms. Yet because the sugar is eaten all day, every day, an allergic reaction to it often goes unsuspected. In fact, sugar addiction is very common. It tastes great so it's fun to eat. And sugar may temporarily make you feel better, giving you a quick burst of energy before you feel the bad effects. Anyhow, it's hard to avoid sugar—it's used in many convenience foods because it's a cheap filler and appeals to all of us with a sweet tooth.

But can you really be allergic to sugar? Many doctors dismiss this as impossible. After all, our bodies naturally convert the carbohydrates we eat into glucose, an essential simple sugar. What these doctors overlook is that the sugar we buy is derived from beets, cane, or corn. A person may react to minute amounts of these foods left in the sugar after the refining process. Double-blind studies have shown that patients believed to be sensitive to cane but not to corn or beets only react to cane sugar when tested, not to corn or beet sugars.[3] Further, because sugar is exposed to gas fumes during processing, a person may be reacting to the gas residues in the sugar.[4]

There are other important reasons for avoiding sugar. Recently, nontraditional allergists have discovered that many allergic people have an overgrowth of yeast in their bodies, which plays havoc with their immune systems (see Chapter 9). Sugar and other carbohydrates feed the yeast, greatly increasing its foothold in the body.

In general, we tend to eat too much sugar. The glucose we need is readily available in many other foods high in carbohydrates, such as vegetables, fruits, or cereals. And, unlike these other carbohydrate sources, sugar contains no protein, vitamins, or minerals. It's empty calories. Even more, by filling up on high-sugar foods, a person may not get enough essential vitamins and minerals, so necessary for fighting off allergies. Too much sugar also interferes with maintaining a stable blood sugar level. Some doctors have observed that although ingesting a large amount of sugar initially makes the blood sugar level rise, it then plunges, causing symptoms of low blood sugar—weakness, nausea, headache, irritability, and mental confusion.[5]

*The Perils of Food Additives.* In thinking about food allergies, don't overlook the chemicals that are often added to enhance commercial products. You may have read in the news about the dangers of food additives such as artificial colorings and flavorings—about their questionable safety and their link to hyperactivity in children. A few years ago, in *Why Your Child Is Hyperactive,* Ben Feingold proposed that in some children hyperactivity is an "intolerance" (not an allergy, since the mechanism is not known) to these additives. Dr. Feingold's claim came as no surprise to many nontraditional doctors, for as early as the late 1940s they had observed that artificial colorings and flavorings caused reactions in many sensitive people. A variety of scientific studies followed Dr. Feingold's report: Some were inconclusive; others showed that a few children seemed to be affected adversely. Unfortunately, these studies didn't take into account the uniqueness of every hyperactive child. Although some hyperactive children are turned on by dyes, others are equally bothered by sugar, milk, corn, molds, and gas fumes. Just removing the dyes from the diet is not enough in many cases.[6]

**Environmental Chemicals**

Sensitivity to the many chemicals in our environment has long been overlooked as a cause of diverse physical and psychological problems. Its mechanism is even less understood than food allergy, but that doesn't mean it doesn't exist.

The thousands of new chemicals synthesized in the last century have seemingly revolutionized our lives for the better, but many doctors are becoming concerned about the effects of these chemicals on our health. Some chemicals are already known to cause cancer and avoiding them is difficult enough. Checking all new and old chemicals for their cancerous potential seems an impossible task. We seem to be constantly bombarded with reports of new carcinogens. It's all too easy to shrug off this information by saying: "Well, nothing's safe anymore. If I'm going to get cancer I'm going to get cancer. I might as well enjoy life now. Why worry about contaminated cranberries, saccharin, cyclamates, beer, cigarettes, or hair dyes? They're bound to find a cancer cure one of these days."

But it isn't only the long-term effects of these chemicals that are worrisome. Nontraditional allergists are concerned because many of their patients seem "allergic" to twentieth-century life. Daily they see patients with all sorts of symptoms brought on by exposure to chemicals in the environment. They believe that these patients are only the tip of the iceberg. The contamination of the environment may well increase as the search for new sources of energy and new chemicals accelerates.

Today, people who are sensitive to the local drinking water can buy (at great expense and inconvenience) spring water. But what will happen when chemically sensitive people need to buy their own air? Actually, for some people, that day is already here. Life in the twentieth century may have many advantages, but the price may be higher than we realize for many, many people.

Offending chemicals are found in our air, water, and foods. They enter the body by way of the mouth, nose, or direct contact with the skin. Some chemicals are present in our environment because we deliberately put them there. Others are beyond our control. For example, in using a room deodorant to mask unpleasant odors you may unknowingly be making yourself sick. Or you may react to air pollution from a factory or auto exhaust. Chlorine is deliberately added to water to kill bacteria, but allergic reactions to it are not uncommon. Inadvertent pollutants in your water supply—insecticides, fertilizers, industrial wastes—may also cause reactions. I've already mentioned food additives—chemicals that are deliberately added to your foods for some specific purpose, such as prolonging shelf life, improving appearance, strengthening flavor, or adding nutrition. Generally, their presence is known because they're listed among the ingredients. Other chemicals (contaminants) accidentally find their way into your food supply. You don't realize they're there.

Unfortunately, most chemically sensitive persons are bothered by more than a single chemical. And you tend to be sensitive to those chemicals to which you're frequently exposed, in the home and workplace. As with food allergies, you may be addicted to the very chemicals that make you sick. Exposure to these chemicals may temporarily make you feel better and repeated exposures seem necessary to maintain your well-being. So you end up craving the offending chemicals. Or, as with food allergies, you may intensely dislike their odor. That's easier.

## ■ A RECONSIDERATION OF RECOGNIZED MEDICAL PROBLEMS

In taking a broad view of allergies, nontraditional allergists have begun to reexamine certain medical problems. They have found that a sensitivity to inhalants, foods, or chemicals may exacerbate or even lie at the root of some common medical disorders.[7] Again, all these syndromes need to be carefully checked out with a physician. But allergy may be an added—and important—factor.

### Alcoholism

Some nontraditional allergists view many alcoholics as victims of an addictive allergic disease. They have found that alcoholics are often allergic to the ingredients in alcoholic beverages. As with other addictive allergies, what happens is that alcoholics feel better when they drink. So the moment they feel they're "crashing" they have another drink. One clue to this is alcoholics' tendency to prefer one drink over another to get their specific fix. If they're sensitive to a particular ingredient, that may be the reason for their craving. A wine drinker, for instance, may be sensitive to grapes, sugar, or brewer's yeast. A beer or bourbon drinker may be reacting to corn, malt, sugar, or brewer's yeast. The rum drinker may be hooked on sugar cane. When reformed alcoholics give up drinking, they may continue to experience intense cravings for alcohol unless they also give up those foods they're sensitive to. In other words, the wine drinker allergic to grapes must give up not only wine but grapes in all forms to feel free of his or her cravings.

**Obesity**

Some overweight people may also be fighting an allergy problem with their favorite foods. Again, the cravings are so strong they can't resist indulging themselves. Eating does make them feel better, at least temporarily. Here another problem is that hunger or thirst itself may be an allergic symptom. One man sensitive to wheat always complained of hunger following a meal high in wheat (pizza, spaghetti, and bread). Thirty minutes after eating such a dinner, he felt "starved" and proceeded to eat a sandwich to ease the hunger pangs. He wasn't really hungry—just experiencing an allergic reaction! Understanding why a person craves a food and why he or she feels so hungry is the first step. Identifying the problem foods is the next.

**Diabetes and Hypoglycemia**

Nontraditional allergists have also observed that some diabetics and hypoglycemics are food allergy victims. Identifying the offending foods can greatly improve their blood sugar problems. It was found that hypoglycemic and diabetic patients in environmental hospital units respectively showed a large decrease or increase in their blood sugar levels when offending foods were returned to their diets after a fast.[8] Avoiding these foods helped to control their symptoms. Some diabetics were even able to reduce their insulin intake with close medical supervision.

High-carbohydrate foods are not the only ones that can cause these blood sugar fluctuations. Doctors have demonstrated that high-protein foods and chemical exposure can cause the same reactions. So a diabetic or hypoglycemic may improve on a low-carbohydrate diet if those are the foods he or she is sensitive to. But if some protein food is the problem, eating a high-protein diet that includes the offending food may make the person worse.[9]

Evaluation of blood sugar levels can also be problematic. Sensitivities to corn sugars, dyes, and flavorings may lead to an abnormal reading on the glucose tolerance test, which is used to diagnose diabetes and hypoglycemia. A person who develops physical or mental symptoms during the glucose tolerance test may simply be reacting to some of the test materials.

### Arthritis

Some victims of arthritis (both osteoarthritis and rheumatoid arthritis) are actually suffering from allergies. Allergies may also lie behind joint pain and stiffness or muscle spasms when all tests for inflammation are negative. The culprits may be foods, chemicals, or inhalants. If some days or seasons are worse than others for pain, redness, and stiffness, this may help pinpoint the allergens.

No place has the relationship of allergy to arthritis been shown more dramatically than in environmentally controlled hospital units (see Chapter 7). Patients suspected of having allergies fast on nothing but spring water for about five days. Often by the end of the fast, pain and stiffness have improved significantly or disappeared altogether—only to reappear when offending foods, chemicals, and inhalants are reintroduced into the diet and environment.

Aside from allergies, toxins in certain foods may cause arthritis in some individuals. Specifically, plants belonging to the nightshade family (tomatoes, potatoes, peppers, eggplants, and tobacco) contain solanine and other poisons which seem to cause a toxic—not an allergic—reaction. Improvement may require from three to 12 months of careful avoidance of these foods.

### Headaches

Many types of headaches—including migraine, sinus, and tension—may be caused by allergic reactions. Awareness is the key. What substances were you exposed to before the onset of the headache? Keeping an Exposure Diary (see Chapter 5) should help you pinpoint what brings on your headaches.

Certain foods in particular have been implicated as frequent triggers of migraine or migraine-type headaches. These are foods containing tyramine (e.g., chocolate and aged cheeses), nitrate preservatives (ham, hot dogs, and cold cuts), monosodium glutamate or MSG (a flavor enhancer found in many prepared and prepackaged foods, as well as virtually all Chinese foods), and excessive salt (most snack foods and many canned soups and vegetables). Alcoholic beverages, especially beer and red wines, are additional offenders. Exactly why these foods provoke headaches in some people is not fully understood yet.

Nonfood triggers of migraine headaches include birth control pills, extreme weather changes, smoke-filled rooms, overly strenuous exercise, loud noises, menstruation, and fluorescent, glaring, or bright lighting. A sensitivity to pollens, molds, dust, and chemical fumes may also cause chronic headaches and migraines.

### Psychological Problems

Most doctors (including both allergists and psychiatrists) scoff at the idea that what we eat, drink, and breathe can dramatically affect our behavior. Nontraditional allergists, however, see allergy as a very frequent cause of mental problems ("cerebral" allergy). Reactions may range from slight depression to Dr. Jekyll-Mr. Hyde personality changes, from a "spaced-out" feeling to schizophrenia, or from mild anxiety to paranoia. Hyperactivity and learning difficulties may appear in children.

Allergies may distort your perception of yourself and your world. If one day you feel really good about yourself and the next you want to crawl under a rock, you may be reacting to something in your environment. If one moment the sun is shining and the next the world goes topsy-turvy, for no obvious reason, ask yourself what you might be reacting to. One day, for example, I started out in good spirits. Then I took Jack to the dentist's office—a chemical environment that always leaves me tired and "down." On the way home we had car trouble and stopped at the gas station, where they put us up on a lift for 30 minutes. The petroleum fumes made me spacey and sleepy. The last straw was walking into a house full of melted plastic fumes from a malfunctioning vacuum cleaner. By evening, I felt awful—exhausted, irritable, weepy, and very depressed. Certainly the car trouble and broken vacuum cleaner were a nuisance, but they were in the realm of minor, everyday frustrations. The real problem was my exposure to all those chemicals. Allergy medicine soon perked me up. By the next day I was fine again.

Behavior problems can also be allergic reactions. Several years ago Jeff began to delight in slugging Jack. First, we attributed it to sibling rivalry. Then we noticed Jeff hit Jack only after eating an apple. During special allergy testing for apples, Jeff's only interest was hitting Jack. When treated for his apple allergy, Jeff's hitting problem immediately disappeared! Amazing? Yes, to most of us—but not to nontraditional allergists, who repeatedly see patients with severe emotional and behavioral problems that improve or disappear after allergy treatment.

It isn't only what we eat. What we don't eat can also cause mental problems. Some nontraditional doctors report great success in treating allergic, as well as nonallergic, patients with large doses of vitamins and minerals. Medical guidance, however, is essential in using large doses of vitamins and minerals since what works for one person may not be the answer for another.

## WHO ARE THESE ALLERGY DETECTIVES?

Having read about this new, expanded view of allergy, you may wonder: Who are these nontraditional doctors who are so concerned about the effects of air, water, food, and chemicals on their patients' health? Many are *clinical ecologists*—medical doctors interested in the effects of the environment on our health. The Society for Clinical Ecology was formed in 1965 by several doctors who felt that allergists' concerns were too narrow. Today, the society has several hundred members. Many became interested in clinical ecology because they themselves or members of their families had health problems that were not being helped by traditional medicine. Once their personal interest was aroused, they began to apply what they learned to help their patients, with considerable success. These clinical ecologists include doctors who are general practitioners, urologists, gynecologists, pediatricians, psychiatrists, surgeons, and allergists.

Other doctors are also interested in environmental medicine. Some ear, nose, and throat specialists look for dietary and environmental factors as well as traditional medical disorders. Orthomolecular physicians are working with allergies, environmental control, and vitamins and minerals to help their patients. They believe that infectious and degenerative diseases can be treated by varying the number of "right" molecules normally found in the body. (The term *orthomolecular,* coined by Nobel Prize winner Linus Pauling, means "pertaining to the right molecule.") Holistic physicians are particularly interested in *all* the influences on a person's health—environment, diet, stress, exercise, and spiritual well-being. Some dentists have also become concerned about their patients' diets and nutrient levels.

Interest in environmentally oriented medicine is not new. As early as the 1920s Albert Rowe used strict diets to help patients with typical allergy symptoms. He also found that patients with other complaints, such as headaches and fatigue, improved on these diets. During the 1930s Herbert Rinkel put forward the concept of hidden or masked food allergies—after testing out his own reactions to eggs. In the 1940s Theron Randolph observed patients who were sensitive to foods and chemicals. After these patients fasted, consuming nothing but spring water for five days, their symptoms often disappeared. Yet when the offending foods or chemicals were reintroduced, their symptoms returned. Later, in 1954, pediatric allergist Frederick Speer coined the term *allergic–tension–fatigue syndrome* to describe a wide variety of symptoms that were not normally recognized as allergy-related.

How to identify allergies was a problem. Arthur Coca discovered why skin tests were not reliable indicators of food allergy: Not everyone with food allergies had the necessary blood chemicals (reagins) to react when food antigens were scratched on the skin. Some new technique was needed. Lawrence Dickey and Guy Pfeiffer discovered that when they dropped a minute extract of the suspected culprit under the patient's tongue, where it was quickly absorbed, symptoms would appear almost immediately if the patient was sensitive. Then Carleton Lee began experimenting with injections of different dilutions of the same extract. He observed that one dose of an extract could provoke symptoms, but another dose of the same extract, at a different strength, could totally relieve symptoms. All this led to the development of provocative testing and neutralization treatment (see Chapter 7).

Today, dietary and environmental changes are recommended by a variety of professionals. Some probation officers, for instance, have indicated that people don't get into trouble if they feel good about themselves—and they can't feel good about themselves if they're constantly tired, achy, or whatever. Dietary and environmental changes (eliminating junk food and sugar, promoting whole grains and extra nutrients, identifying and treating excess toxic metals in the body) have helped some prisoners in jail or on probation feel so much better that they've turned their mixed-up lives around and become responsible citizens. As another example: Some counselors for couples experiencing marital problems have found that the difficulties are more easily resolved once diets and environments are changed. If both partners feel better about themselves, they're more likely to feel better about each other.

How influential allergies, dietary inadequacies, and a polluted environment are on many of our social problems is of course debatable. Yet there are those who believe that our diets (which are drastically different from our ancestors' diets), coupled with environmental pollution, contribute to many of our social problems—including divorce, drug abuse, crime, juvenile delinquency, alcoholism, child abuse, violence, and learning difficulties.[10] They are trying to make the public more aware of the relationship between environment and behavior and good health.

# SECTION TWO

# You and Your Allergies

# 3

## Are *You* Allergic?

How can you find out if allergies might be causing your symptoms?* First, of course, you need to go to your doctor for a complete physical. But if the cause of your symptoms remains unexplained and no treatment seems to work, you might consider consulting a clinical ecologist or some other doctor interested in the effects of the environment on your health. What can you expect?

To begin with, a nontraditional allergist would ask you questions like those found in this and later chapters—to determine if you do indeed have allergies and, if so, what substances should be suspected as the culprits. If you're curious, why not try asking yourself some of these questions now? Several affirmative answers should make you *suspect* allergies. But it's definitely advisable to check this out with an expert.

### ■ FAMILY MEDICAL HISTORY

1. Do any blood relatives (parents, grandparents, aunts, uncles, siblings, and children) suffer from:
   —Traditionally recognized allergy syndromes (hay fever or allergic rhinitis, asthma, skin rashes, or severe reactions to drugs or insect stings)?
   —Food allergies?

*See Chart 1, pages 59–63, for a list of symptoms and their suspected allergens.

—Addictive disorders such as compulsive eating, alcoholism, or drug abuse? Are any blood relatives "sugarholics"?
—Diabetes or low blood sugar?
—Arthritis, headaches, digestive disorders, or other diseases and symptoms listed in Chapter 2?

2. Were any relatives hyperactive, learning-disabled, or bed wetters as children?

## PERSONAL MEDICAL HISTORY

### Infancy

1. Did your mother experience severe stress while she was pregnant with you? Was your birth difficult? Were there any complications? (Stress before, during, or after birth may contribute to allergic problems.)
2. If you were breast-fed, did you have any problems with gaining weight, colic, or spitting up? (If yes, you may have been sensitive to foods your mother was eating that entered her milk in minute amounts.)
3. If you were bottle-fed, were there difficulties in tolerating your formula or problems with gaining weight, colic, spitting up, or vomiting? (If yes, you may have been sensitive to cow's milk or some other ingredient in the formula.)
4. Did you have frequent health problems? Was there trouble with:
   —Digestion (colic, gas, diarrhea, stomachaches, or frequent spitting up or vomiting)?
   —Respiratory and related ailments (stuffy nose, noisy breathing, frequent ear infections)?
   —Eczema or other skin rashes?
5. Have you been described as a "difficult" baby? As an irritable, fussy baby who cried a lot? As one with sleeping problems? As overactive?

**Childhood**

1. Did you have any traditionally recognized allergy problems, such as asthma or hives?
2. Were you often sick, plagued by:
   —Ear infections, sore throats, swollen glands, colds, bronchitis, or croup?
   —Stomachaches, constipation, or diarrhea?
   —Headaches?
3. Did you have other seemingly inexplicable symptoms, such as:
   —Recurrent leg or muscle aches?
   —Always feeling exhausted despite sufficient sleep?
   —Dark circles under your eyes?
   —A pale, washed-out complexion even though blood tests for anemia were normal?
   —A frequently itchy or stuffy nose?
4. Was bed-wetting a problem after age three?
5. What about behavior problems? Were you irritable? Overactive or underactive? Did you have a short attention span or trouble learning in school?
6. Were you a problem eater?

**Adulthood**

1. Do you suffer from any traditionally recognized allergy syndromes, or is there anything you already know you're allergic to?
2. Are you always coming down with colds or some kind of "bug"?
3. Have you been troubled by various somatic complaints, such as:
   —Frequent digestive upsets, gas or belching, bouts of constipation or diarrhea?
   —Sinus problems, postnasal drip, earaches, recurrent sore throats?
   —Repeated bladder infections, difficulty urinating, water retention?

—Headaches, dizziness, convulsions?
—Leg or muscle aches, back pain, swollen or stiff joints, arthritis?
—A constant low-grade fever, feeling flushed or chilled, excessive sweating, fainting spells?

4. Are you always tired, even though you get enough sleep? When you wake up in the morning, do you feel exhausted?
5. Is something "not quite right" about your appearance? Can you see dark circles under your eyes? Is your complexion pale? Do you look or feel puffy? Bloated?
6. What about eating difficulties? Do any foods make you sick? Are you a picky eater? A binger?
7. Do you feel like a yo-yo? Are you high one moment, low the next? Do you get depressed for no reason?
8. Is your activity level a problem? Do you have trouble concentrating, or sometimes feel confused and spacey? Or is it more the opposite? Are you hyperactive, overly nervous, or frequently anxious?
9. Do your symptoms come and go? Are they worse one day but better the next? More acute in one season than another?
10. Does a change in yoiur surroundings change how you feel? Are things different if you're at home or at work?
11. Have you already noticed shifts in how you feel, depending on what you're doing or what's going on around you? Are certain odors, for instance, irritating, even when they don't bother other people? Does stress make your symptoms worse?

# 4

# What Are *You* Allergic To?

So you think you may have allergies. It's time to begin some detective work. How can you determine which substances bother you? Inhalants, foods, and chemicals—these are the three major types of offenders. And within each area, there are a number of possible criminals. To help you along in unmasking the culprits, this chapter includes a variety of questions similar to those a clinical ecologist might ask you. In answering these questions, you may want to keep a "detective's" notebook—listing all the substances that arouse suspicions. (This may also be helpful if you later visit a clinical ecologist, as a start for his or her culprit hunting.) A "yes" response to any question should alert you to the possibility of a sensitivity.

## INHALANT OFFENDERS

### House Dust

The fine gray powder that results from the natural deterioration of such household items as mattresses, carpeting, curtains, papers, books, and clothes—that's house dust. Another component is the house-dust mite, a microscopic spiderlike bug that is found wherever people are, especially in bedding and mattresses.

House dust is what you see floating, seemingly suspended, on sunbeams indoors. It's what you throw away when you empty your vacuum cleaner. Dust settles everywhere, and it accumulates in areas that aren't frequently cleaned. But even the best-kept houses have house dust in the air.

*Questions to Ask*

1. Do your symptoms occur year-round but especially in the fall and winter months when the furnace constantly blows dust throughout the house? Is there an improvement when you go outside?
2. Do you feel worse when you vacuum or clean the house? Are your symptoms more acute when you empty the vacuum cleaner or dust with a cloth or mop? Does your nose begin to itch or run?
3. When you make a trip to the attic or a dusty library, are your symptoms worse?

**Molds**

Molds belong to the group of plants called fungi, which have no true roots, stems, leaves, flowers, or green pigment and which reproduce by means of spores. You're probably familiar with the furry mold that grows on old bread or leftover food. There are thousands of different types of molds. They are found all over the world, in soil, air, and water; they flourish in damp, dark areas, both inside and outside.

The weather affects the molds in the air you breathe in. Rainfall, high humidity, and wind disperse mold spores, making the mold-sensitive person miserable. Molds tend to grow best in cool temperatures, without direct sunlight. Night air thus contains more spores than day. Although the air is never free of mold spores, in the winter, when the ground is frozen and covered by snow, they are less prevalent outdoors.

Molds are also present in certain foods, such as some cheeses. Persons who are mold-sensitive are frequently sensitive to other members of the fungi family—baker's yeast (raised baked goods), brewer's yeast (alcoholic beverages, vinegar, B-vitamin preparations, and enriched foods), and mushrooms.

*Questions to Ask*

1. Do your symptoms come on or get worse during the mold seasons in your area (usually the spring or fall months)? And are they better during the winter if the ground is frozen and snow-covered? If you live in a farming region, are your symptoms acute during grain-harvesting season?
2. Does damp, windy weather make your symptoms worse? Have you noticed any increase an hour before or after a rain storm?
3. Is there a change for the worse at night?
4. Does raking leaves, cutting grass, or working with your hands in the soil aggravate your symptoms?
5. When you're in a damp and musty-smelling house, do your symptoms improve if you leave but get worse if you return?
6. If you work in an area where molds thrive (for instance, a library, bakery, cheese factory, farm, greenhouse, grain storage area, tanning factory, saw or textile mill), are your symptoms worse at work and better at home, on weekends, or during vacations?
7. Are you susceptible to fungus infections like thrush mouth, athlete's foot, ringworm, skin or vaginal yeast infections?
8. Do you react to baker's yeast, brewer's yeast, or mushrooms?
9. Are you sensitive to antibiotics made from molds, such as penicillin?

**Pollens**

Pollens are the yellow, powderlike particles found on flowers. Heavy, sticky pollens are usually not a problem because they don't become airborne, but lighter pollens are easily carried by the wind, sometimes hundreds of miles. Fortunately, only a comparatively small number of these tend to be allergenic. The most common problem-causing pollens come from certain trees, grasses, and weeds. Ragweed is a well-known example.

The pollen season will depend on where you live. Your newspaper or TV and radio weather reports may give the pollen count for your area. This pollen count represents the number of grains of a specified variety of pollen (usually ragweed) present in a given volume of air at a specified time and place. Following these reports may help you correlate these pollens with your symptoms. Pollen seasons often overlap with high mold counts, but pollen-producing plants are killed by the first frost while high mold counts continue until snow or freezing temperatures arrive.

*Questions to Ask*

1. Do your symptoms begin or get worse during your local pollen season? Are they worst on days with the highest pollen counts?
2. Is there a decrease or disappearance of symptoms with the first frost?
3. During the pollen season do you feel better in an air-conditioned indoor setting than outdoors?
4. Does a hard, continuous rain bring relief during high-pollen months? And are windy days the worst?
5. In the pollen season are your symptoms aggravated by such activities as cutting the grass, weeding the garden, or picnicking in the countryside?
6. Are your symptoms worse during the month or two preceding the appearance of all the leaves on your trees? If so, you may be sensitive to tree pollens.

**Animal Danders and Hairs**

Any animal with fur or feathers can provoke allergic symptoms in sensitive people. Common culprits are cats, dogs, horses, rabbits, mice, hamsters, gerbils, parakeets, cattle, hogs, sheep, goats and chickens. Contact with live animals isn't the only offender, however. Feathers in pillows, sleeping bags, quilts, comforters, or furniture may bring on symptoms. So may exposure to animal fur or hair found in common articles such as wool clothing, fur-lined gloves, or chairs and mattresses padded with horse hair. Remember: You may be sensitive to one kind of animal dander and not another.

*Questions to Ask*

1. Are your symptoms aggravated by contact with a furry or feathered animal? Did your symptoms start or increase when you got a new pet?
2. Does contact with animal fur or hair in clothes or furniture make your symptoms worse? If you sleep on a feather pillow, for instance, do you wake up with symptoms? Have you found that wearing wool makes you itch or break out?
3. If you work with animals (e.g., farmer, veterinarian, or petshop owner), are your symptoms worse at work?
4. When you visit a zoo or petshop, do your symptoms increase?

## ■ FOOD CULPRITS

Checking out food allergies may seem an overwhelming task—there are so many possibilities. First, you need to find out whether you should suspect some food or foods as a cause of your symptoms. If you answer "yes" to several of the following questions, one or more food allergies may be at the root of your problems.

1. Are you already aware that certain foods make you sick?
2. Do you feel worse after eating? Is your nose stuffy after a snack or meal? Are you plagued by bloating, belching, or indigestion after meals? Sleepiness?
3. Do you feel better if you skip meals or fast?
4. If you don't eat on time, do you feel weak, disoriented, or irritable? And do you feel better after eating? Have you been diagnosed as hypoglycemic (having low blood sugar)?
5. Are you a picky eater? Do you hate certain foods?
6. Is binging a problem? Do you crave certain foods? Are you overweight, with a family or personal history of allergy?
7. Do you frequently get mouth ulcers or canker sores? Does your tongue look like a map (geographic tongue)? Is bad breath a problem?
8. Are you troubled by bouts of diarrhea or constipation?
9. Have you ever had stomach ulcers?
10. Do you often feel puffy? Does it seem you easily gain weight, even though you're not overeating?
11. Are you or have you ever been a bed wetter?
12. Do alcoholic beverages make you feel worse? Better? Do you experience side effects with even a small amount of alcohol? Are you hung over after just one drink?

Now, if you've begun to suspect food allergy, you'll want to hunt out the possible offenders. As a first step, try making the following lists:

—Foods you already know make you sick.

—Special cravings. Is there something you *have* to eat every day? What food, if you ran out of it, would make you go to the store at any hour of the day?
—Foods you dislike.
—Any food whose smell or cooking aroma makes you sick.

The next step is to narrow down your list of suspects. Here are some questions that may help you rout out two of the most common culprits—milk and sugar:

1. As a baby, did you have trouble with colic, frequent spitting up, skin rashes, eczema, or frequent ear infections? Has there ever been any time in your life when you could not drink milk because it made you sick? Do any blood relatives avoid milk because it makes them sick? Do you crave or hate milk, cheese, yogurt, ice cream, or creamed foods? Are you only satisfied if you drink more than 16 ounces of milk a day? Is cream in your coffee a must? If you've answered "yes" to several questions, suspect *milk.*
2. Do you crave sweets, soft drinks, pastries, or alcoholic beverages? Is sugar in your coffee crucial? Does eating sugar temporarily make you feel better? Do you ever eat sugar just by itself? This time if you've answered "yes," suspect *sugar.*

Now let's explore your food cravings. What is it that you *have* to have? Is it:

—Chocolate? Suspect *chocolate* and *sugar.* Also suspect related foods such as *coffee* and *cola* beverages.
—Coffee? If you have to have your cup of coffee

every day or drink more than two cups a day, suspect *coffee*.

—Popcorn, corn-on-the-cob, corn chips, corn cereal, or soft drinks sweetened with corn syrup? Suspect *corn*.

—Corn-distilled liquors such as bourbon? Suspect *corn, sugar,* and *yeast*.

—Wine? Suspect *grapes, yeast,* and *sugar*.

—Pastries, breads, and pasta? Suspect *wheat*.

—Pizza, spaghetti, and catsup? Suspect *tomatoes*.

—Peanuts, peanut butter, peanut butter cookies, or candy containing peanuts? Suspect *peanuts*.

—Oranges, orange juice, orange sherbet, or anything orange-flavored? Suspect *oranges*.

—Applesauce, apple pie, or raw apples? Suspect *apples*.

—Apple pie, spice cake, cinnamon toast, or cinnamon-flavored gum? Suspect *cinnamon* and *sugar*.

Sometimes symptoms are worse around certain holidays because you eat more of certain foods that bother you. Ask yourself if any particular holiday aggravates your symptoms. Do you feel worse around:

—Valentine's Day? Suspect *corn, sugar, chocolate, nuts*, and *red dye*.

—Easter? Suspect *sugar, corn, chocolate, nuts, artificial colorings and flavorings*, and *eggs*.

—Halloween? Suspect *corn, sugar, chocolate, nuts, artificial colorings and flavorings, apples*, and *cinnamon*.

—Christmas? Suspect *sugar, corn, chocolate, nuts, artificial colorings and flavorings*, and *alcoholic beverages*.

—Birthdays? Suspect *sugar, wheat, artificial color-*

*ings and flavorings, chocolate, milk,* and *soy* (used in icings).

Here are a few more suggestions for tracking down your food allergies. If there's a seasonal pattern to your symptoms, you may be reacting to certain seasonal foods such as strawberries, melons, or turkey. How about different types of cuisine? Does eating Italian food often cause symptoms? Perhaps you're sensitive to tomatoes, wheat, milk, or the seasonings. Finally, consider that you may react to some foods only if you eat large portions of them; you may tolerate smaller amounts eaten infrequently.

## ■ CHEMICAL TROUBLEMAKERS

How do you know if you're chemically sensitive? Again, awareness is the key. You need to observe where and when you start to experience symptoms and note what you have been exposed to at the time. As a beginning step, try answering the following general questions:

1. Have you ever been exposed to massive amounts of toxic chemicals?
2. Are you frequently exposed to toxic chemicals at work, home, or while pursuing hobbies? Did your symptoms begin or get worse after starting a new job, buying a new home, or becoming involved in a new hobby?
3. Are you more *or* less aware of chemical odors (particularly natural gas leaks) than other people?
4. Do you crave the smell of certain chemicals that others find offensive? Or is it the opposite: Do you hate the smell of certain chemicals that others find

pleasant or inoffensive? Will you go out of your way to smell certain chemicals?

5. Are your symptoms worse when you're driving in traffic, or in an area of high air pollution? Do you feel better in clean air areas—at the oceanside, in the country, or high in the mountains?
6. Have you observed mood changes during certain activities? For instance, are your symptoms aggravated by shopping trips, in crowds, or at social gatherings?

If you think you are chemically sensitive, you may wonder how you can single out possible offenders from the thousands of chemicals in your environment. The following information and questions may help you make a list of suspicious chemicals.

### Cleaning Chemicals

Ironically, cleaning products, which are designed to remove unwanted substances, contain a variety of potentially offensive chemicals. Thus, keeping the indoor environment clean can be a perplexing job for the allergic person. You will need to keep your home as free from dust and mold as possible if you have inhalant allergies. But you may *also* be sensitive to your cleaning products. Even if you don't clean the house yourself, the odor of cleaning chemicals will linger. It's very difficult, sometimes impossible, to remove the odors of certain agents once they've been used.

*Questions to Ask*

1. Do your symptoms become worse when you use:
   —Chlorine (found in bleach, scrubbing cleansers, deodorizers, disinfectants, and swimming pools)?
   —Ammonia (found in glass cleaners, bathroom cleansers, and oven cleaners)?

—Furniture polish?
—Floor wax?
—Scented soaps, detergents, cleansers, and fabric softeners?
—Carbon tetrachloride or spot removers?
—Products for rug care such as detergents, soil retardants, deodorizers, shampoos, and spot removers?

2. Do you especially enjoy or dislike the odors of any cleaning products? Will you go out of your way to sniff them?
3. Have you noticed that your symptoms become worse when you're in the aisle of your grocery store with all the cleaning products? Again, do you find their odor very pleasant or irritating?

**Cosmetics, Perfumes, and Other Personal Care Products**

Many people suffering from cosmetic allergies are unaware of the source of their symptoms. They don't think that something as everyday as their soap or skin cream could be causing problems. With more men using various cosmetics, they too are suffering from reactions to their own cosmetics, as well as to those used by other men and women. How many marriages are unhappy because his aftershave makes her depressed and her perfume makes him sleepy?

But even those who suspect they're sensitive may overlook some potential offenders. There is no such thing, for instance, as a nonallergenic cosmetic. There is always someone who will react to one of the ingredients. The term *hypo-allergenic* simply means *less* allergenic, not *nonallergenic*. Hypo-allergenic cosmetics supposedly exclude the 60 ingredients found to commonly cause allergic reactions. But government testing of all products is impossible; moreover, it is difficult for government and industry to agree on standards for hypo-allergenic products. The Food and Drug Administration allows a company to claim a product is hypo-allergenic for two and a half years before the company must substantiate this claim with evidence. So the label *hypo-allergenic* may not be very helpful to the chemically sensitive person.

Perfumes or fragrances present a number of hidden dangers for the chemically sensitive. With expensive perfumes it may be easier to identify the problem sources, as they are usually pure oil extracts from rare flowers. Inexpensive perfumes and scents used in cosmetics, however, are a different story, for they are rarely pure. You may react to any one (or several) of their typical ingredients: flower oil, plant leaves, needles, roots, animal substances, synthetic chemicals from petroleum or coal tar, phenol and alcohol. And there are many, many products containing fragrances, including toilet papers, facial tissues, lipsticks, body deodorants, aftershave lotions, shaving creams, soaps, shampoos, hair sprays, room deodorizers, and candles.

Besides fragrances, cosmetics may contain other problem ingredients—natural or synthetic. Two potent natural allergens are orrisroot and karaya gum, found in some toothpastes, shaving creams, skin creams, suntan lotions, shampoos, lipsticks, hair preparations, soaps, and perfumes. Other natural ingredients often causing problems are cornstarch, acacia or gum arabic, olive oil, pine oil and scent, cottonseed, lanolin, and potato starch. Two potent synthetic allergens still commonly found in cosmetics are paraben esters and ethylene diamine. They are also used in drugs to treat your skin problems, often compounding the original rash. Other synthetic chemicals frequently causing reactions are azo dyes, phenol, ethers, mineral oil, petroleum jelly, Formalin (formaldehyde), creosol, and various alcohols. Yet another often unsuspected source of cosmetics allergy comes from the mold and bacteria that may grow freely in such products as eye shadow and liquid makeup.

*Questions to Ask*

1. Can you relate the onset of your symptoms to the use of any cosmetics? Have you noticed any change in symptoms if you switch brands of cosmetics or scented products, or if you don't wear makeup?
2. Do you crave the smell of any of your own cosmetics or other scented products?
3. If your spouse uses scented cosmetics, are your symptoms worse when you're close to him or her?
4. Do your symptoms increase in crowds, at church, social gatherings, beauty salons, or barber shops? Is the cosmetics counter a danger area?
5. When you use a room deodorant, does it aggravate your symptoms?
6. If you use scented tampons or sanitary napkins, are your symptoms worse during your periods?

**Drugs**

Americans live in a drug-oriented society. We are constantly bombarded by advertisements telling us that "relief is just a swallow away." With waiting rooms full of patients demanding instant cure, some harassed doctors may end up writing prescriptions even when a patient's illness would go away by itself and medication is unnecessary. Some patients aren't satisfied without a pill. Yet drugs may end up causing more illness than they relieve, especially with the chemically susceptible patient.

Prescription drugs aren't the only offenders. Don't overlook aspirin, vitamins, or any other over-the-counter medication as a possible cause of symptoms. Even seemingly innocuous products such as throat lozenges and sprays or mouthwashes may contain phenol, artificial colorings and flavorings, or sugar.

Chemically sensitive people may react to the drug itself or to such fillers and coloring agents as:

—Cornstarch (a frequent ingredient in drugs from aspirin to vitamins).
—Milk derivatives such as lactose (milk sugar) and calcium lactate (both commonly used as binders and fillers in tablets and capsules).
—Brewer's yeast (commonly found in B-vitamin preparations).
—Coal tar dyes (routinely used as colorings to make identification easier and to make preparations more eye-appealing).
—Artificial flavorings (often used to make medications more palatable).
—Sugar (cane or beet) or artificial sweeteners (used as fillers or to make the medicine taste better).

*Questions to Ask*

1. Did any of your current symptoms begin or get worse after you started taking any drug (either prescribed or over-the-counter)?
2. Are there any ingredients you know you're sensitive to in your current drugs? (Check for fillers, colorings, or flavorings.)
3. Do you crave any of the drugs you take?
4. Have you had to take more and more of a certain drug to get the same effect?

### Fabrics

With fabrics, you may be sensitve to the fibers themselves or to the chemicals with which the cloth is processed. A few people are sensitive to natural fibers (wool, cotton, silk, and linen) or to their finishing chemicals, but more people are bothered by synthetics. Not only are clothes a problem, but so are sheets, blankets, drapes, carpets, and upholstery.

Both natural and synthetic fabrics are usually treated with a variety of chemicals through dying, sizing, Scotchgarding, sanitizing, permanent pressing (formaldehyde), and mothproofing (pesticides). Labels are not very helpful because they don't indicate what chemicals have been used in the processing. Trying to identify the offending chemicals can be a very frustrating task.

*Questions to Ask*

1. Do your symptoms become worse:
   —In a fabric or furniture store?
   —When you're trying on new clothes?
   —If you sew new fabrics?
   —With new upholstery or carpeting?
2. Is the touch or smell of certain fabrics offensive?

**Formaldehyde**

You may think formaldehyde is only used in biology labs to preserve dead specimens and thus isn't a problem for you. Unfortunately, formaldehyde is widely used. There may be high levels of it in the air in your home, school, or office without your being aware of its presence. Whether you inhale formaldehyde or absorb it through the skin, it can cause severe problems if you are sensitive to it.

Recently, urea-formaldehyde foam insulation has been banned because it emits too much formaldehyde, which has cancer-causing properties. But once foam insulation has been installed, it's very difficult to remove. Formaldehyde gas continues to be slowly released into the air; high temperatures and high humidity increase this. Nor is insulation the only culprit. Formaldehyde is widely used in building supplies such as particle board, paneling, concrete, plaster, wallboard, wood veneers, and synthetic resins. New buildings are made to be as airtight as possible to conserve energy, so the formaldehyde may not have a chance to "gas out"; often outside air doesn't circulate freely inside and windows can't be opened.

New carpeting, upholstered furniture, and drapes may also give off formaldehyde fumes. Personal care products such as nail polishes, nail hardeners, mouthwashes, toothpastes, antiperspirants, soaps, and shampoos may contain "Formalin" (a mix of formaldehyde and alcohol). In paper products, formaldehyde is used to improve wet strength. Some medications contain formaldehyde as a preservative, and it is found in some insecticides.

Formaldehyde forms naturally in coal, wood, and tobacco smoke, and it is one of the important, irritating pollutants in smog. As if all this weren't enough, formaldehyde is used to make maple sap run more freely so there may even be traces in your "pure" maple syrup!

*Questions to Ask*

1. Have you already listed yourself as sensitive to other chemicals? (If so, you may well be sensitive to formaldehyde as it's contained in so many products.)
2. Do your symptoms get worse:
   —In households with urea-formaldehyde foam insulation?
   —Inside a mobile home or camper, where particle board, wood veneers, carpeting, or drapes may emit formaldehyde and the air may not circulate freely?
   —In fabric or clothing stores, rug shops, or furniture stores?

—When you're exposed to unfinished particle board or plywood?
—With a wood-burning stove?
—In a smoke-filled room?
—With cosmetics containing Formalin?

3. Can you date the start of your symptoms to buying a new house, or new carpeting, drapes, or furniture?
4. If your symptoms seem worse at work, are you frequently exposed to sources of formaldehyde on your job? Is your work area new and tightly insulated?

### Newsprint, Inks, and Office Supplies

Modern offices are often "the pits" for chemically sensitive employees. Not only do carpeting, furniture, and paneling emit noxious fumes in rooms with poor ventilation, but the very tools of the trade—glue, pens, tape, paper, carbon paper, newsprint, and copying machines—may be bothersome. Of course, you don't have to work in an office to use these products frequently.

*Questions to Ask*

1. Have you noticed that your symptoms get worse when you do office work?
2. Are your symptoms triggered by the smell of fresh newsprint or the odors of ink, carbon paper, typewriter ribbons, stencils, and copying machines? Do you crave any of these smells?
3. Does a visit to a printer or copying shop spoil your day?

### Paints

The odor from paints is a common troublemaker for the chemically sensitive person. Fresh paint is the worst, but odors may linger for some time. Also, some paints may be more offensive than others.

*Questions to Ask*

1. Do you find the odor of paints very pleasant or extremely irritating?
2. When you enter a newly painted room, do your symptoms get worse?

**Pesticides**

Even if you follow all the directions on the labels, using pesticides may make your life miserable. And even if you don't use pesticides yourself, you may be exposed to their effects. Since World War II, pesticides have been used more and more in schools, workplaces, and outdoors. They're routinely used in grocery stores, florists, orchards, farms, warehouses, factories, apartments, motels, and mosquito-control projects. Once pesticides have been used, it's extremely difficult (if not impossible) to get rid of the residues.

*Questions to Ask*

1. Are you attracted to or disgusted by the odor of mothballs, insect repellants, or weed-killers? And does using them bring on symptoms?
2. Have you noticed a reaction after exterminators have treated your house or if you use pesticides yourself?
3. If pesticides are routinely used in your workplace, are your symptoms worse at work and better at home or on vacation?
4. Do your symptoms get worse in grocery stores, greenhouses, florists, or other places where pesticides may be used?
5. Are your symptoms aggravated when mosquito-control trucks spray pesticides in your neighborhood?

**Petroleum Products and Gas Fumes**

Petroleum products and gas fumes are a major source of symptoms for the chemically sensitive person. Every facet of modern life means exposure to these chemicals in one form or another. Obvious sources are gasoline, oil, tar, diesel fuel, and home heating oil. But petrochemicals are widely used in making drugs, artificial food colorings and flavorings, clothing dyes, plastics, cleaning agents, cosmetics, fabrics, and pesticides. The list is endless, and so are the problems caused.

*Questions to Ask*

1. Do you love to smell gasoline and associate its odor with a feeling of well-being, or do you hate the aroma and try to avoid it? Are your symptoms worse in gas stations? When you use a gasoline-powered lawn mower?
2. Have you noticed an increase in symptoms when you're driving a car or riding in a bus? Do you get carsick or sleepy? If you're behind a smelly bus or truck, does this aggravate symptoms? Is standing on the corner in an area of heavy traffic an invitation to symptoms?
3. If you have a gas or oil furnace, do you feel worse in the winter when the furnace is running?
4. If you have a gas stove, do you often feel sick in the kitchen, whether the stove is on or not? Have you experienced symptoms when cooking?
5. Are your symptoms worse around any other gas sources, such as gas or kerosene heaters, gas-lit fireplaces, or gas dryers?
6. Does mineral oil taken as a laxative make you sick? What about mineral oil in lotions, cold creams, and cosmetics?

7. Does the odor or application of petroleum jelly products aggravate your symptoms?
8. Do you like, dislike, or are you made sick by the odors from:
   —Floor waxes, glass wax, furniture polish, or burning wax candles?
   —Machine oils used in typewriters, sewing machines, or other appliances?
   —Lighter fluids?
   —Nail polish or nail polish remover?
   —Newly dry-cleaned fabrics?
   —Recently manufactured plastics, such as new shower curtains or placemats, or a new car?

### Phenol (Carbolic Acid)

Another common offender is phenol, or carbolic acid. This organic chemical is widely used in disinfectants, cosmetics, plastics, and pesticides. It may even be present in allergy treatment extracts!

*Questions to Ask*

1. Do you find the odor of phenol-containing disinfectants very pleasant or very irritating, or does it make you sick?
2. When you get a whiff of disinfectants in public restrooms, do symptoms develop?
3. Have you found you cannot tolerate allergy injections or other injections containing phenol as a preservative?
4. Are symptoms brought on by using phenol-containing throat lozenges or sprays, or mouthwashes?

### Pine

Not all chemical reactions are provoked by synthetic materials. The odor of pine, for instance, can make some sensitive people ill, particularly those with petrochemical intolerances. Our current supply of oil and coal is believed to be derived from prehistoric pine forests, so this relationship seems reasonable.

*Questions to Ask*

1. Do you crave, hate, or are you made ill by the smell of evergreen decorations, burning pine logs, or pine cones?
2. Are your symptoms worse during the Christmas season, and especially near a Christmas tree?
3. Do you feel worse in a room paneled with pine?
4. Have you noticed that using pine- or cedar-scented deodorants, soaps, bath oils, shampoos, disinfectants, or furniture polishes brings on symptoms? Does turpentine aggravate your symptoms?

**Tobacco**

Smoke from cigarettes, cigars, or pipes is an extremely common source of symptoms for the chemically susceptible person. It's not just the tobacco itself that causes the problems, but all the chemicals used in the growing, curing, and processing.

*Questions to Ask*

1. If you are otherwise chemically sensitive, have you ever smoked or do you smoke now? Are you frequently exposed to tobacco smoke?
2. Do you find tobacco smells either very pleasant or quite offensive?
3. Are your symptoms worse in places where people are smoking?

**Water**

If you're chemically sensitive, you may react to drinking water that contains chlorine, fluoride, or other chemicals. Chlorine is deliberately added to water in very small amounts for purification, but it may also be a potent allergen. Fluoride may be added to decrease tooth decay, or it may occur naturally. Pesticides and other organic chemicals may enter the water supply from runoffs from agricultural areas, chemical dumping grounds, or industrial sewage-disposal sites.

*Questions to Ask*

1. Are your symptoms better when you vacation in an area with spring or well water but worse when you return home to chlorinated water?
2. Do your symptoms increase around chlorinated swimming pools, when you use chlorine bleach, or if you fill the tub with chlorinated water?
3. Do you find the taste of your drinking water very offensive?
4. Is your water supply known to be contaminated with chemicals?

## ■ AN ADDITIONAL GUIDE

To double-check or expand your list of suspected substances, you may want to look over the following chart, which shows some of the most common substances causing particular allergy symptoms. This chart, however, is only an abbreviated guideline. Also keep in mind that just about any substance can cause just about any symptom in any person.

**CHART 1. Guide to Suspected Allergens**

| *Symptoms* | *Area of Suspected Sensitivity* | *Possible Specific Offenders* |
|---|---|---|
| Alcoholism | Foods | Sugar, corn, brewer's yeast, barley, grapes |
| Anaphylaxis | Foods | Eggs, fish, shellfish, nuts |
| | Drugs | Penicillin |
| | Insect stings | Bees, wasps, yellow jackets, hornets |
| Behavior problems (especially hyperactivity or learning disorders) | Inhalants | Dust, mold, pollen |
| | Foods | Sugar, milk, corn, chocolate, wheat, eggs, citrus |
| | Food additives | Artificial colorings and flavorings, preservatives (BHA, BHT, nitrites) |
| | Chemicals | Petrochemicals, formaldehyde, chlorine, perfume, inks, paint fumes, tobacco, cleaning chemicals |
| Blood-sugar disorders (diabetes or hypoglycemia) | Foods | Both low- and high-carbohydrate foods (cheese, meat, fruit, sugar) |
| | Chemicals | Petrochemicals |

**CHART 1. Guide to Suspected Allergens *(continued)***

| *Symptoms* | *Area of Suspected Sensitivity* | *Possible Specific Offenders* |
|---|---|---|
| Cardiovascular disturbances (high blood pressure, irregular heartbeat, angina) | Inhalants | Mold |
| | Foods | Corn, chocolate, nuts, coffee, milk, wheat, beef, pork, seafood, apples |
| | Chemicals | Petrochemicals, formaldehyde, odor of soft plastics, perfume, tobacco, pesticides |
| Digestive disturbances | | |
| *In infants:* Colic, formula problems, frequent spitting up | Foods | Formula (milk, soy, corn, sugar) |
| | | Vitamin drops (artificial colorings and flavorings, corn syrup, sugar, cod liver oil) |
| | | Breast milk (foods eaten by mother) |
| | | Solid foods (wheat, rice, oats, barley) |
| *In children and adults:* Indigestion, heartburn, nausea, vomiting, gas, colitis, constipation, diarrhea, gallbladder pain, hemorrhoids, stomach ulcer, etc. | Foods | Milk, wheat, eggs, corn, nuts, chocolate, orange, pork, beef, chicken, sugar |
| | Food additives | Preservatives |
| | Chemicals | Petrochemicals, chlorine |

| | | |
|---|---|---|
| Canker sores | Foods | Citrus, pickles, apples, coffee, chocolate, potatoes, nuts, cinnamon |
| Ear, nose, or throat problems (ear infections, frequent colds, runny nose, hay fever, coughing, sneezing, nosebleeds, tonsillitis, sinusitis, nasal polyps, etc.) | Inhalants | Dust, mold, pollen, animal dander |
| | Foods | Milk, eggs, chocolate, peanuts, corn, wheat, chicken, oranges |
| | Food additives | Artificial colorings |
| | Chemicals | Petrochemicals |
| Headaches (migraine and other types) | Inhalants | Dust, mold, pollen |
| | Foods | Chocolate, aged cheese, milk, citrus, alcoholic beverages |
| | Food additives | Nitrites, MSG (monosodium glutamate) |
| | Chemicals | Petrochemicals, tobacco, perfume, cleaning agents, paint fumes |
| Mental difficulties (anxiety, depression, poor memory or concentration, "brain fag," irritability, etc.) | Inhalants | Dust, mold |
| | Foods | Sugar, milk, wheat, corn, rye, chocolate |
| | Food additives | Artificial colorings and flavorings, preservatives (BHA and BHT) |
| | Chemicals | Petrochemicals, formaldehyde, chlorine, tobacco, perfume, paint fumes |

**CHART 1. Guide to Suspected Allergens *(continued)***

| *Symptoms* | *Area of Suspected Sensitivity* | *Possible Specific Offenders* |
|---|---|---|
| Muscle or joint discomfort (muscle spasms, cramps, weakness, joint pain and stiffness, arthritis, etc.) | Inhalants | Mold |
| | Foods | Milk, chocolate, wheat, beef, pork, chicken, coffee, eggs, sugar |
| | Food Additives | Artificial colorings, preservatives |
| | Chemicals | Petrochemicals, tobacco, chlorine |
| Respiratory ailments (wheezing, asthma) | Inhalants | Dust, mold, pollen, animal dander |
| | Foods | Milk, eggs, grains, corn, fish, shellfish, peanuts, chocolate, nuts, onions, garlic |
| | Food additives | Artificial coloring |
| | Chemicals | Tobacco, petrochemicals, formaldehyde, chlorine, perfume, paint fumes, cleaning agents |
| | Drugs | Aspirin |
| Seizures | Foods | Milk, yeast, chicken |
| | Chemicals | Petrochemicals, formaldehyde |
| Skin problems | | |
| Contact dermatitis | Chemicals | Cosmetics, metals in jewelry, industrial chemicals |
| | Plants | Poison ivy and oak |

| | | |
|---|---|---|
| Hives | Foods | Chocolate, milk, eggs, peanuts, cinnamon; also seasonal foods like strawberries, melons, tomatoes |
| | Food additives | Preservatives, artificial colorings and flavorings |
| | Drugs | Aspirin, pencillin |
| Eczema | Inhalants | Dust, mold, pollen, animal dander |
| | Foods | Milk, chocolate, nuts, peanuts, eggs |
| Urinary difficulties (bladder infections, painful and frequent urination, bed-wetting, etc.) | Inhalants | Mold |
| | Foods | Milk, eggs, citrus, tomatoes, corn, wheat, pork, chicken, cola, chocolate, onions, fish, cinnamon, apples, peanuts |
| | Food additives | Artificial colorings, preservatives |
| | Chemicals | Tobacco |

# 5

# Self-Help Steps to Track Down *Your* Allergies

Now you have a list of allergenic substances that may be causing your symptoms. This chapter will help you expand your list and confirm your observations. Then consult Chapters 6 and 7 for avoidance and treatment measures.

## EXPOSURE DIARY

Begin by keeping a diary for a week or more, noting the time of day of each exposure to inhalants, foods, beverages, and chemicals. Don't forget drugs, toothpaste, and other personal care products. Record the weather. Write down all your physical and mental symptoms.

Before exposure to a particular substance or activity ask yourself: "How do I feel? Do I hurt any place? Am I tired? Is my nose itchy or runny? Am I okay mentally or am I spacey, confused, or depressed?" Ask yourself the same questions after each exposure. Are you the same, better, or worse? You may want to use a number scale to indicate how bad your reactions are, with 5 as severe and 1 as symptom-free. If you're housecleaning, for instance, record how you feel before, which cleaning products you use, what you clean, and how you feel afterwards. Learn to listen to what your body is telling you.

After you've completed your Exposure Diary, answer these questions: "Are there days when I feel good and other days when I don't? What is *different* on the bad days? What allergens was I exposed to on the bad days that I wasn't exposed to on good days?" Add these possible culprits to your list if they are not already there.

Now you want to confirm the suspicious items on your list. Unfortunately, there's not much you can do to confirm *inhalant* allergies on your own except continue to note your exposures and any reactions. If these seem consistent, you're ready to start a program for avoiding the offending substances as much as possible (see Chapter 6). If your symptoms are severe or chronic, you should find an interested doctor who can confirm your suspicions and recommend treatment in addition to avoidance measures (see Chapter 7).

If your symptoms are not severe or chronic and you do not have such symptoms as depression, diabetes, heart trouble, or epilepsy, you might try the steps below to check your food and chemical sensitivities. *If in doubt, always consult your doctor first.*

## ■ TRACKING DOWN FOOD ALLERGIES*

First, you have to confirm *which* foods cause problems. Then, you have to determine *how much* food, if any, can be tolerated and *how frequently.* You also need to learn how long it takes you to react to a food after you've eaten it. Some people react immediately; others don't react for several hours, or even longer.

---

*This material was excerpted and adapted from William G. Crook, M.D.: *Tracking Down Hidden Food Allergies.*

There are several different ways to detect food sensitivities. Select the method that's easiest for you. Don't reintroduce foods whose very odor makes you ill. Never reintroduce a food that has caused a severe reaction such as a swollen tongue, hives, asthma, collapse, or shock—unless you are under the care of an experienced doctor.

**The Elimination Diet**

On an elimination diet you exclude a given food (or foods) from your diet for seven to eight days, or until your symptoms have improved for two days. You may not be symptom-free, but you should feel better. Then, you reintroduce each food in pure form, one food at a time, and note your symptoms. If you feel worse when a food is returned to your diet, that food becomes suspect.

When you allow a week between eating the food and then reintroducing it, your reaction will be more exaggerated than if you ate the food every day. If, however, the food is withheld too long, you may develop some tolerance to it and not react to it the first few times you eat it. So you don't think it's a suspect and begin to include it again in your diet. What happens is that you become sensitized again, but you go on eating the culprit food because you seemed okay on its initial reintroduction. *The timing of an elimination diet is very important.*

How do you begin? Take your list of suspected foods. Add these to a Common Foods Elimination Diet, which cuts out the following commonly eaten foods: milk, chocolate, cola, coffee, corn, eggs, citrus, sugar, wheat, and rye. Food additives, even though they are really chemicals, should be included, so artificial colorings and flavorings are to be avoided. This diet is outlined with menus in Appendix A. Chapters 14 to 20 supply safe recipes and will help you adapt your own recipes to the restrictions of your diet.

The advantage of combining your own suspect foods with the Common Foods Elimination Diet is that it saves you time. You'll soon learn what your trouble sources are. If, however, you find this diet too restrictive or too hard to follow, you may want to try only one food or a few foods at a time.

Before going through a step-by-step account, let's get a general picture of what an elimination diet is like. Suppose you're trying an elimination diet for milk, sugar, and chocolate. Remember to keep a careful Exposure Diary throughout. Begin by eating all three foods—you might try homemade chocolate milk or ice cream made from milk, cocoa, and sugar. Then avoid milk, sugar, and chocolate in any form for one week. At first you may feel worse and your symptoms may be exaggerated. You may have strong cravings for those foods. Hang in! It'll be worth it.

Now it's the eighth day. You test for milk by drinking pure milk as often as you like, starting at breakfast. If by lunchtime you feel tired, irritable, depressed, achy, or your nose is stopped up, milk becomes a number one suspect. Once again you stop drinking it in all forms.

Now you wait until the milk reaction subsides (24 to 48 hours) before testing for sugar. Let's say on the tenth day you are feeling better. So you eat some pure sugar cubes or add sugar to unsweetened pineapple juice or grape juice. By midmorning you're in the pits and your legs ache. Sugar is added to your list of suspicious foods. Again, you wait until the sugar reaction has subsided before going on to chocolate.

By the twelfth day you're feeling better. Now you return to chocolate in pure form. You are still avoiding milk and sugar. At lunchtime you're still feeling good so you eat some more pure chocolate. Again, no reaction. After eating pure chocolate once again later in the day and experiencing no symptoms, you conclude that chocolate is not a problem for you.

What do you do now? You avoid milk and sugar totally for one to two months. Then you see if you can tolerate small amounts, eaten once every four or five days.

Keep in mind, however, that you may have several food allergies—say, to milk *and* citrus. If you eliminate only milk, you may drink more orange juice, causing symptoms. On the other hand, if you go on a citrus-free diet, you may drink more milk, believing it's okay. You end up still having symptoms. So you draw the wrong conclusion—thinking that neither milk nor citrus is a problem.

A *Step-by-Step Guide.* Now let's go through the Common Foods Elimination Diet step by step. The same principles apply to any elimination diet. Don't forget to keep your Exposure Diary.

1. *Initial Testing:* Eat the foods to be tested before starting the diet. Your body must be exposed to each food before it is withdrawn.
2. *Abstinence Period:* The trial elimination period should last seven to eight days, or until the symptoms have subsided for two days. During this time avoid the foods you're testing in all forms. Don't worry if you feel worse at first—your body is just telling you it wants another fix. Stick with it!
3. *Reintroducing the Foods:* After a week, begin to reintroduce the foods into your diet, one at a time, in pure form—starting at breakfast. Begin with the food you least suspect. Save your favorite food for last.
4. *How to Serve a Pure Food:* Obviously, you don't

want to reintroduce several foods that have been mixed together because then you won't know which one causes the reaction. Ice cream, for example, contains milk, sugar, artificial colorings, and eggs. So how do you make sure you eat a pure form? Here are some suggestions:

—*Milk:* A glass of plain milk.

—*Sugar:* Sugar cubes or granulated sugar in unsweetened pineapple juice. (If you usually eat both cane and beet sugar, you must test each separately.)

—*Chocolate:* A bar of unsweetened chocolate or pure cocoa powder mixed with water.

—*Coffee:* The coffee you regularly drink but without cream or sugar.

—*Citrus:* A fresh orange in sections or fresh-squeezed orange juice.

—*Eggs:* A hard- or soft-boiled egg or scrambled eggs (without milk), cooked in pure safflower or sunflower oil.

—*Wheat:* Cream of wheat but without milk or sugar.

—*Rye:* Plain rye crackers.

—*Artificial colorings:* Mix together equal amounts of food colors, then add a half-teaspoon of that mixture to unsweetened pineapple or grape juice.

—*Corn:* Corn-on-the-cob with safflower margarine or plain popcorn cooked in pure corn oil (no butter).

5. *How to Read Your Initial Reactions:* If you don't get a reaction the first time the food is served, eat the food again at a midmorning snack or lunch—still in pure form. Keep eating this food all day, or until symptoms develop. Once you observe symptoms, stop eating the food. If no symptoms are provoked

by bedtime and you've followed the diet carefully, you can assume that you're not sensitive to that food. Keep that food out of your diet, however, while you test the other foods.

6. *Reintroducing Another Food:* If you react to a food, wait until the reaction subsides (24 to 48 hours) before reintroducing the next food. If there is no reaction, you can return another food to your diet the next day. But only test one food at a time.
7. *What to Do about Bad Reactions:* Your doctor may recommend one of the following if you suffer a bad reaction: unflavored milk of magnesia, Alka-Seltzer Gold (aspirin-free), a half-teaspoon of baking soda in 16 ounces of water, vitamin C, or an antihistamine.

*Some Additional Pointers.* When you go on an elimination diet, *be sure to read all labels carefully.* The common foods are often found in food mixtures, so if the contents of a package aren't listed, don't buy it. Unfortunately, even reading the labels isn't a guarantee, as there are several problems with current food labels. First, they may not fully disclose the ingredients. A manufacturer may list *vegetable oil,* for instance, without disclosing the fact that the oil used contains a preservative like BHA or BHT. The term *butter* does not tell you if the butter used was already colored. In other words, the ingredients of ingredients are often not listed. Sometimes you have no way of knowing which oil or mixture of oils was used—soy, corn, cottonseed, coconut, or peanut. The oils used in a product will vary according to their current price levels. So one time you may eat a food with no reaction and another time you may react—because a different oil was used. Another problem is that sometimes the packaging material is treated with preservatives that leech into the food, but these preservatives are not listed among the ingredients.

Don't be deceived by labels that flaunt the terms *pure, natural, 100% natural* or *all natural* in large print. A careful reading of the fine print may reveal artificial ingredients like colorings, flavorings, and preservatives. Also, remember that sugar and corn sweeteners are considered natural ingredients.

And not all products have labels. Ice cream, cheese, and butter, for instance, do not have to list ingredients. They have a "standard of identity" set by the government.

So how can you tell if a product is okay for you to eat? About all you can do is to read labels carefully. When in doubt, contact the manufacturer. Many companies are very helpful. If you're still in doubt after corresponding with them, avoid the product.

Another tip for your elimination diet: *Be sure to plan your menus before you start.* You don't want to discover when you go to fix dinner that you don't have the necessary supplies to stay on the diet. Also, when you're away from home, take a "safe" snack along. If you break the diet, you have to start all over again, so try to do it right the first time! Even one little bite or swallow of a forebidden food during the diet may distort the results. If you crave forbidden foods, it's best to keep them out of the house until the day you return them to your diet. Don't cheat or you may not learn anything. Good planning will save you much time and effort.

Start looking for or making staples you'll need before you start your diet. Recipes for catsup, mayonnaise, mustard, and other staples are included in Chapter 14. You'll also need to buy sugar-free and corn-free salt, corn-free baking powder, rice and oat flours, and pure honey. Try to obtain color-free and flavor-free drugs if any must be taken. Don't use toothpaste; it contains colorings, flavorings, and corn. Instead, brush with sea salt and baking soda. Don't use mouthwash.

*How to Evaluate Your Reactions.* What symptoms should you watch for when you reintroduce a food? Any symptoms are possible, but here are some of the most common—headaches, a runny nose, dark circles under the eyes, a rash, itching, stomachaches, joint pains and stiffness, overactivity, irritability, depression, and fatigue. These symptoms can be confusing; they may not be the ones you usually experience. For instance, if joint pain is your major problem, you may be surprised when your nose starts to run after a food is returned to your diet. Even if your joints don't flare up, you should regard your runny nose as a sign that the food bothers you and is contributing to your joint problems. Any adverse reaction means that food is contributing to your problems and must be avoided.

If you're not sure about a food after going through an elimination diet, then repeat that food elimination diet. You don't want to eliminate a nutritious food if you aren't sensitive to it, but you don't want to overlook any problem either.

What if you don't feel better on the elimination diet after ten days? Try returning all at once, in excess, all the foods being tested. If you don't feel worse when all these foods are eaten, you're probably not sensitive to them. If you do feel worse, repeat the elimination diet, reintroducing the foods one at a time.

Finally, what if you feel worse on the elimination diet? This clue should make you suspect foods you are substituting for the ones eliminated. Try an elimination diet with these new suspects.

**Tips for Specific Elimination Diets**

If you don't use the Common Foods Elimination Diet, you can try eliminating specific foods or food groups, in any order. Here are some pointers for each diet.

*Chocolate, Cocoa, Cola, and Coffee*. Chocolate, cocoa, cola, and coffee all belong to the same food family, so a sensitivity to one may mean a sensitivity to other family members. Of course, there are good reasons (caffeine and sugar) to avoid these foods in any case, but if you suspect you're sensitive, then try an elimination diet.

The first few days may be really rough, for these foods can be very addictive. You may have better success if you gradually decrease the amount you're consuming over a week or two, and then remove these foods totally from your diet. Herb teas may help replace coffee. Postum, a coffee substitute, contains wheat, malt, and molasses (cane sugar). Substitute pure carob powder for chocolate and cocoa (see Chapter 19 for recipes).

*Cane and Beet Sugars.* Labels on sugar bags or boxes may not state whether the sugar is cane or beet. Which one is used will depend on where you live and the current price of each sugar. If you use both cane and beet sugars, you should test each separately. Beets should also be avoided on a beet sugar elimination diet.

It's hard to cut out all sugar because it's found everywhere. Catsup, barbecue sauce, pickles, mayonnaise, hot dogs, table salt, liquor, corn syrup, and maple syrup—these are just some of the less obvious places. Be sure to read all labels carefully. The following ingredients mean cane or beet sugar may be present:

—Sucrose
—Natural sweetener
—Confectioners' sugar
—Turbinado sugar
—Brown sugar
—Molasses
—Raw sugar
—Cane

You may substitute pure honey and pure maple syrup for sugar in recipes (for examples and suggestions, see Chapter 15).

A note of caution: Withdrawal symptoms from sugar can be severe. If you are a sugar addict, you should cut down the amount you're eating before you try a sugar elimination.

*Artificial Colorings.* Artificial colorings are found in many prepared foods such as cake mixes, butter, cheese, ice cream, crackers, soups, hot dogs, pastries, and jams. Read labels carefully, looking for the following:

—U.S. certified colors
—Artificial colors added
—Yellow dye (or whatever color)
—FD & C colors

If the label states: "Natural color added," it should be okay.

*Milk.* Cow's milk is the most common food allergen in the United States. On this elimination diet, cow's milk and goat's milk should be avoided in all forms. Milk is often found in breads, soups, margarines, powdered artificial sweetners, so-called nondairy creamers, cereals, luncheon meats, vegetables with butter or milk sauces, and dessert mixes, to name just a few. When reading labels, watch out for the following terms, which may mean *milk:*

—Nonfat dried milk solids
—Evaporated milk
—Condensed milk

—Lactose
—Whey
—Cream
—Cheese
—Butter
—Margarine
—Casein
—Calcium caseinate
—Sodium caseinate
—Lactalbumin
—Curds
—Yogurt
—Lactate

Both adults and children can survive quite well without milk for the duration of a milk elimination diet. Although milk supplies protein, phosphorus and vitamins A, D, and $B_{12}$, these nutrients are available elsewhere. You will want to supplement your diet with calcium if you must avoid milk on a long-term basis.

*Corn.* Corn rivals milk for the top spot on the list of allergy-causing foods. Corn is widely used in many forms. It is commonly found in table salt, confectioners' sugar, chewing gum, baking powder, margarine, catsup, pickles, cereals, sweetened fruit juices, fruits packed in syrup, hot dogs, luncheon meats, mixed vegetables, soups, and vitamins. The glucose used in the glucose tolerance test has a corn base, so a sensitivity to corn may confuse the test results. Corn may also be found in nonfood items like toothpaste, aspirin, many medications, cough syrup, bath powders, stamps, gummed labels, envelopes, and paper cups—just to name a few! The following ingredients suggest corn may present:

—Syrup
—Cornstarch
—Starch
—Hominy
—Grits
—Sugar
—Corn sweeteners
—Sweeteners
—Malt
—Dextrose
—Dextrine
—Glucose
—Fructose
—Shortening

—Vegetable oil
—Maize
—Bourbon

For a corn elimination diet, you will need to locate a corn-free baking powder, or you can easily make your own (see Chapter 18). You will also need to use pure vegetable oil, such as safflower or sunflower, for cooking, and a corn-free margarine.

*Wheat and Rye.* Some people are sensitive to all grains (wheat, rye, oats, barley, and rice), but sometimes if one grain isn't tolerated others can be. On this diet, you should avoid wheat, barley, and rye, which are closely related, as well as all grain-distilled liquors. You may eat oats, rice, and nongrain starches such as tapioca, potato, soy, arrowroot, or pure buckwheat. Remember, however, that commercial rye, potato, and oat breads almost always contain wheat flour. When reading labels watch for the following ingredients:

—Flour
—Wheat flour
—Wholewheat flour
—Wheat germ
—Graham flour
—Bran
—Durum flour
—Semolina
—Gluten flour
—Enriched flour
—Monosodium glutamate (MSG)

*Eggs.* Avoid both egg whites and egg yolks on an egg elimination diet. Eggs are commonly found in baked goods, clarified coffee, noodles, root beer, some breads, mayonnaise, tartar sauce, ice cream, and some egg-substitute products. They are also found in live vaccines for polio, mumps, and measles. Some terms indicating the presence of eggs in a product are:

—Vitellin
—Globulin
—Ovomucin
—Albumin
—Egg whites
—Egg yolks
—Powdered eggs
—Dried eggs
—Whole eggs

*Citrus.* Fruits to avoid on this diet are oranges, - grapefruits, ugli fruit, lemons, limes, kumquats, and tangerines. You do not need to eliminate citric acid. Test those citrus fruits you eat frequently. Sometimes even if one citrus fruit is not tolerated, others may be.

If you must avoid all citrus after the elimination diet, you will want to be sure you're getting enough vitamin C in your diet, as this vitamin is often obtained from eating citrus fruits. Other good sources of vitamin C are cantaloupe, tomato, guava, mango, papaya, broccoli, Brussels sprouts, and green pepper. You may need to take vitamin C tablets to ensure a daily supply.

*Other Common Troublemakers.* Tomatoes and apples often present problems. Also common is a sensitivity to one or more members of the legume family—peas, green beans, carob, peanuts, and soybeans. Soy is particularly difficult to avoid as it is found everywhere—in shortenings, baked goods, vitamins, breads, mayonnaise, salad dressings, and infant formulas. Lecithin and food "extenders" are soy derivatives.

Cinnamon, a frequent troublemaker, is widely used in many baked goods. In trying a cinnamon-free diet, avoid any product that just lists "spices" on the label. If you're sensitive to cinnamon, try substituting allspice, which is not related but has a similar taste.

By now you may be shaking your head in total confusion and wondering what you'll ever be able to eat. Take heart! Once you've tried an elimination diet, you'll find it's not all that difficult. But don't expect to accomplish all this overnight. It takes a while to track down problem foods and to learn to listen to what your body and mind are telling you.

### The Caveman Diet

The Caveman Diet is another kind of elimination diet. It eliminates every food you eat more than once a week. Here are the allowed foods:

—Rarely eaten fresh or frozen fruits and vegetables
—Meats, poultry (wild game, if possible), and fish
—Sea salt
—Water (distilled or mineral)

These foods should be fresh, if at all possible; frozen, if necessary. If canned, they must be unsweetened or canned in their own juices or water. The meats and fish must be pure—no breading, smoking, or curing allowed (as in ham, bacon, hot dogs, or luncheon meats). Try to find fish, poultry, and meat you do not usually eat. Dairy products, cereal grains, sugar, spices, and herbs are not permitted.

After a week on this diet, you should be feeling better. Return eliminated foods to your diet, one per day, in large amounts. Note any reactions.

### Fasting

Fasting is another alternative method to determine which foods, if any, are causing your symptoms. Fasting isn't for everyone. *Don't fast unless your doctor gives an okay.* Diabetics, epileptics, asthmatics, and those with heart disease, severe dizziness, kidney disease, or severe depression should fast *only* under their doctor's close supervision.

During a fast you should drink only pure spring water stored in glass containers and eat nothing for five to seven days. When you feel hungry, drink spring water instead. Drinking lots of spring water throughout the fast will help rid the body of toxic wastes. Don't smoke. (You may find that fasting helps you kick the habit more easily than any other method.) Some doctors have their patients continue their vitamins and minerals during the fast; others do not. If possible, all medications should be stopped—but check with your doctor first. Taking unflavored milk of magnesia at the beginning of the fast and every other day helps to rid your system of foods and chemicals.

Try to control your chemical exposures as much as possible during the fast. Before you start, remove as many chemical products from your house as possible. Don't use toothpaste, cosmetics, hair spray, or perfume during the fast.

You may experience withdrawal symptoms the first few days and feel worse than before. Don't panic. This is a good sign; it means your body misses some of the foods that have been causing your symptoms. A half-teaspoon of baking soda in 16 ounces of water helps to relieve symptoms. (If your symptoms are extremely severe and nothing seems to help, you can always break the fast and start eating again.) You should, however, start to feel much better by the fourth day or so of the fast, with a clearing of your symptoms and an increase in energy. Keep a careful Exposure Diary.

After five to seven days, add back your foods—one at a time, allowing at least several hours between foods. Start with those foods you least suspect. If, after eating a food, you still feel well, several hours later you can add another food. If you have a reaction, don't try another food until you're feeling good again. You should end up with a list of foods that cause symptoms and another list of well-tolerated foods. From these lists, you can make a rotation diet (described in Chapter 6).

## ■ TRACKING DOWN SENSITIVITIES TO CHEMICALS IN FOOD

Can you guess what product is made with the following ingredients?

> Water, corn syrup, flour, animal fat (with BHA, BHT, propyl gallate, and citric acid), sugar, graham flour, dextrose, corn flour, whey solids, food starch, gelatin, mono and diglycerides, salt, banana flakes, cellulose gum, molasses, trisodium phosphate, honey, baking soda, polysorbate 60, artificial flavor, vanilla, artificial color (FD & C Yellow No. 5).

It's banana cream pie!

Tracking down hidden food allergies is difficult enough, but the chemicals added to foods complicate the task. Some of these chemicals *(food additives)* are deliberately put in for some specific purpose—to prolong shelf life, improve appearance or flavor, or enrich nutrition. Their presence is easily determined because they're usually listed among the ingredients. Other chemicals *(food contaminants)* accidentally find their way into the food supply. The consumer doesn't realize they're there. For the chemically susceptible person, these chemicals may play a major role in disease.

Not all additives are bad for you. But it's difficult for concerned consumers to know which additives may cause problems for them, which ones have been poorly tested for safety, and which ones are harmless or even beneficial.

Part of the problem is the unfamiliar technical names. They're so confusing and hard to pronounce, they inspire distrust. And there are so many additives to keep straight. Admittedly, natural foods are also made up of many chemicals with strange names. When we talk of a protein food, for instance, we don't mention which amino acids it contains (e.g., tryptophan, lysine, or histidine). And just because Mother Nature produces a chemical doesn't ensure its safety. For example, a person who is allergic to aspirin may actually be sensitive to salicylate, a chemical found not only in aspirin but also naturally in some fruits and vegetables.

The problem faced by the chemically sensitive person is this: How can you determine whether reactions are caused by the food itself or by one or more chemicals added to it? No one sits down to a bowl of BHT or a plate of red dye, so the real culprits may go unsuspected. If, however, you know you're sensitive to other chemicals, then you should be suspicious about the chemicals in your food if you still have symptoms. Let's say you can eat potato chips prepared in pure soybean oil, but you get sick when you eat potato chips fried in soybean oil with BHT added. You should conclude you're sensitive to BHT.

Here's one way to go about investigating your sensitivity to the chemicals in your foods: First, stock up on a week's worth of organic foods to which you know you're not sensitive. Do you feel better by the end of the week? Then, add back five or six meals of regular foods from the grocery store. Again, these are foods to which you aren't sensitive, but they are probably chemically contaminated. Are your symptoms worse? If you feel better on the organic foods, this may be your only alternative, even though it's expensive, inconvenient, and time-consuming.

For more information about additives and contaminants in your foods, consult Appendix C. If you find the technical names too frustrating and confusing, then follow this general rule: If you can't pronounce the ingredient, don't buy the product!

## ■ TRACKING DOWN CHEMICAL SENSITIVITIES

One way for you to test chemicals at home is to purchase small glass bottles with tight-fitting tops. Test one chemical at a time—and only when you're feeling good. Place a ball of cotton in the bottom. Then, put several drops of the suspected chemical on the cotton. Quickly close the bottle and seal it tightly. Avoid that chemical as much as possible for five days. Then, go back and open the bottle. Take several sniffs and note any reactions. Be sure to keep a careful record of your symptoms before and after the sniff tests. Do not attempt these tests if you have any severe symptoms.

If you know how to check your pulse, you can add this to the sniff test. Before opening the bottle, take your pulse for one full minute. Then, after opening the bottle and taking several sniffs, count your pulse again for one minute, and then again every ten minutes. An increase or decrease in pulse rate of 12 to 20 beats—with or without symptoms—suggests you're sensitive to this chemical.

The sniff test is particularly good for checking out sensitivities to perfumes, hair sprays, formaldehyde, alcohol, furniture polishes, detergents, chlorine bleach, fabric softeners, aftershave lotions, and paints. But *don't try this test when you're by yourself.* And *stop testing as soon as symptoms occur.* If your reaction is severe, try breathing fresh air. Again, doctors often recommend Alka-Seltzer Gold or a half-teaspoon of baking soda in 16 ounces of water.

If you develop symptoms when testing a chemical, you should avoid or reduce future exposures. For avoidance suggestions and medical treatment, consult Chapters 6 and 7.

# 6

# How to Avoid *Your* Allergens

Now you have a list of inhalants, foods, or chemicals that seem to make you sick. What can you do? The cheapest, safest, and most effective treatment for allergies is always *avoidance,* if possible. Even when other treatments are used, avoidance should be part of the total program. Unfortunately, total avoidance is sometimes impossible. You can completely cut out chocolate and tomatoes from your diet, but you can't get rid of *all* the mold in your environment. But don't despair. Any measure that reduces your exposure to an allergen will help lower your total allergic load, thereby reducing symptoms.

## HOW TO MINIMIZE INHALANTS

Although you can't totally remove inhalant particles from the air you breathe in, you can reduce their number. *Electronic air cleaners* remove molds, house dust, and pollens from the air. Because particles in the air are electrically charged, they are attracted to an oppositely charged filter. The filter is then either washed or replaced periodically. The best models use High-Efficiency Particulate Air (HEPA) filters. Some units with charcoal filters also remove chemicals, such as tobacco smoke. Choose an electrostatic air cleaner that produces less than .01 parts per million of ozone gas, for ozone will bother you if you are chemically sensitive. The unit should also remove more than 90% of particles from 10 to .01 microns in size.

There are several different types of air cleaner units. One kind fits on a forced-air heating system. Smaller room units are less expensive and are preferred by some doctors because they can keep one, closed-off room freer of allergens than a central unit can. Suppose you use a smaller unit in your bedroom. Then, for eight hours each night, while you sleep, your air can be well controlled. Of course, in addition to using the air cleaner, you should take extra precautions to make your bedroom as free of dust, mold, and chemicals as possible. Living in a controlled atmosphere for eight hours each day will help you tolerate your exposures the rest of the time.

If possible, rent a room-sized electronic air cleaner for a month to see if you feel better and whether the odor of the unit bothers you. Some chemically susceptible people react to one type of filter but not another. With a doctor's prescription, these units may even be tax-deductible. There are also smaller portable units for traveling and units that work in your car. Beware, however, of the many inexpensive units that advertise scented filters. Even if the machine has a switch to turn off the scent, you may still get enough scent to make you ill if you're chemically sensitive.

Using the right kind of *vacuum cleaner* also helps. The ones with upright bags are the worst because dust passes through the bags back into the air. A cylinder or cannister type is better. More effective vacuums work with water instead of bags; the dust is drawn into the water, which is then discarded. Central vacuum systems are the best (but quite expensive); here the dust is deposited outside the house.

### House Dust

Here are some guidelines for dust-proofing a bedroom:

1. Empty the room. Remove all carpets, rugs, and drapes. Vacuum all parts of the bed. Clean the room thoroughly with a tolerated cleaning solution. Return only essential items. Because carpets and rugs hold dust and mold while giving off chemical fumes, it's best to keep them out.
2. Cover the mattress and box springs with allergen-proof encasings. Don't use plastic ones if you're chemically susceptible.
3. Cover the furnace vent in the room with cheesecloth and change it frequently. Even better, seal off the vents and use an electric heater instead.
4. Dust and vacuum the room daily and give it a thorough cleaning weekly.
5. Keep the room free of dust-catchers, such as books, knick-knacks, toys, and pictures.

Other steps you can take to reduce your exposure to house dust include:

1. Changing your furnace filters frequently.
2. Using an allergy mask while you're cleaning. Or hiring someone to clean your house (it may be well worth the extra money).

### Molds

Remember that molds thrive in cool, damp, and poorly ventilated areas. Here are some ways to reduce the mold population indoors:

1. Clean mold-prone areas frequently with tolerated disinfectants. Refrigerators, refrigerator drip pans, garbage pails, and spaces under sinks are common places where molds thrive.
2. Keep air conditioners, humidifiers, dehumidifiers, and vaporizers scrupulously free of mold, using tolerated cleaning agents.
3. Check behind wallpaper and paneling for mold growth. Also look under carpets and carpet padding, particularly in areas that have been wet or damp. If your house smells moldy, but you can't find the source, examine inside the walls.
4. Keep bathrooms as dry as possible. Use an exhaust fan to circulate fresh air. Scrub tiles and grouting around tubs and showers with tolerated disinfectants. Don't use carpets. Change towels frequently and launder damp towels as soon as possible. Avoid leaving sweaty clothes in the hamper, as they encourage mold growth. Dry your toothbrush after using.
5. Make sure closets, drawers, and hampers are free of damp or perspiration-stained clothing or bedding.
6. Take special care with bedding. Old bedding breeds mold spores. Synthetic pillows discourage mold growth but often bother the chemically sensitive person. Cover pillows and mattresses with allergen-proof encasings.
7. Don't put old clothes, shoes, furs, overstuffed furniture, or leather products in storage areas. Discard old newspapers, books, and magazines.
8. Replace old, overstuffed furniture, which is frequently very moldy inside. Caution, however, is needed if you replace it. Polyester fibers and urethane sponge discourage mold growth but may bother the chemically sensitive person.

9. If you have a damp basement, especially one with a dirt floor, take steps to make it drier. Good ventilation and lighting are essential. A dehumidifier will take moisture out of the air, but be sure to clean it regularly, as the molds thrive in the collected moisture. A sack of calcium chloride suspended over a pail also will absorb moisture. Clean the pail frequently. Seal all basement cracks. Clean all moldy areas with tolerated disinfectants. Paint walls and floors with mold-resistant paints (if tolerated). Throw out old junk.
10. Check any fruits and vegetables stored in a basement or cellar for mold growth.
11. Watch out for houseplants, as they are often a source of mold because of their moist soil. If you aren't willing to part with your plants permanently, ask a friend to keep them temporarily to see if your symptoms improve. In summer keep them outdoors, if possible. Never have houseplants in your bedroom. Crushed rock on top of the soil around each plant will help keep the mold spores from entering the air.
12. Be careful about treating your house with special chemicals like Formalin (formaldehyde) and Zephiran, which kill off molds. These chemicals often bother the chemically susceptible, causing worse problems than molds. Borax in water is a good mold-retardant and is well tolerated.

Reducing your mold exposure outdoors may be even more difficult, but there are steps you can take:

1. Don't rake leaves. Alternaria, Hormodendrum, and Pullularia are molds that thrive on dead leaves.
2. Don't mow the lawn yourself, and stay away while someone else is mowing it. Cutting grass stirs up the

molds, disperses grass pollen in the spring, and exposes you to turpenes (the natural chemicals that give cut grass its odor).
3. Be sure to wear gloves when gardening, as molds thrive in soil.
4. Stay away from compost and hay.
5. Wear an allergy mask to help reduce your mold exposure if you have to do some yard chores yourself.
6. Stay inside on windy days.

**Pollens**

Avoiding pollens during the pollen season may be hard. Still, here are some measures to try:

1. Get weeds and grasses in your yard and adjacent lots cut so that they can't pollinate.
2. Keep away from related allergens. If you're sensitive to ragweed, you're probably also sensitive to marigolds and chrysanthemums. Insect repellents that contain pyrethrum (a chrysanthemum-derivative) may bother you.
3. Stay inside as much as possible during the pollen season. Use an air conditioner and keep windows and doors closed.
4. If you must be outside for a while, wear an allergy mask. But don't participate in such outside activities as golf, picnics, and hayrides.
5. Keep car windows rolled up during pollen season and use an air conditioner.
6. Plan your vacation for the worst weeks of your pollen season. Escape to the mountains or seashore, if possible.

**Animal Danders and Hairs**

Try these suggestions to control your contact with animal danders, hairs, furs, and feathers:

1. If you don't have a pet now, don't get one—unless it's a fish or a reptile! Although not very huggable, these animals won't aggravate your allergies.
2. If you already have a pet who's a beloved family member, *at least* keep the animal out of the bedrooms. Vacuum frequently. Have the pet live outside, if possible. You might ask a friend to keep your pet for a few weeks, to see if your symptoms really do improve.
3. Keep away from farms, stables, zoos, petshops, and similar places.
4. Instead of a feather pillow, try a synthetic one if you're not chemically sensitive. Or stuff pillow cases with *cotton* towels, blankets, or diapers.

## HOW TO CUT OUT FOODS

If you are only sensitive to a few foods, it may be easy to eliminate them by carefully reading labels, staying away from mixtures of foods, asking ingredients when eating out, and using Chapters 14 to 20 to adjust your own recipes. Vary your diet as much as possible to avoid developing more food allergies.

### A Rotation Diet

If you have multiple food allergies, you may need to use a rotation diet. Rotation or rotary diets are used for several purposes: to detect food allergies, to "treat" current food allergies, and to prevent future food sensitivities. A rotation diet systematically varies the food served as much as possible. The farther apart you space your foods the better. Doctors recommend four-day rotation diets for some patients, five-day diets for others, and even longer ones for patients with very severe food allergies.

Chart 2 shows a five-day rotation diet. On the first

day eat any of the foods listed under Day 1, but do not serve any other food. On the second day select only foods listed under Day 2, and so on through Day 5. After the fifth day start over with Day 1. On this diet no food is eaten more often than once every five days. It includes all the major foods and doesn't eliminate any. If you react to any of these foods, even though you eat them only once every five days, you should eliminate them from your diet for several months. Then, see if you can tolerate them once every five days.

To make up your own rotation diet, group together members of the same food family (see Appendix E). Eat these foods on the same day, since they are chemically similar. For instance, asparagus, garlic, leeks, and onions belong to the same family, so they should be served on the same day. Some doctors, however, allow members of the same food family to be eaten on different days, as long as there are two days intervening. For instance, if you eat grapefruit on Monday, then you can eat oranges on Thursday.

In designing your rotation diet use only your safe foods. Avoid your problem foods for several months. If you have severe multiple food allergies, there may be only enough safe foods to eat one per meal, but you may eat as much of that food as you wish. After a while you can try adding more foods to your rotation diet—one at a time. If you still react to a food, eliminate it again for several months.

What would a *very* restricted diet look like? Chart 3 outlines a limited four-day rotation diet for someone who has just finished fasting and has discovered 16 safe foods. This diet may seem very unusual, but you can still feel quite good and satisfied on it. In any case, such restricted rotation diets should only be temporary, although you may have to continue to rotate your foods for some time to avoid symptoms.

**CHART 2. Five-Day Rotation Diet**

| *Type of Food* | *Day 1* | *Day 2* | *Day 3* | *Day 4* | *Day 5* |
|---|---|---|---|---|---|
| Meat, fish, poultry | Chicken, eggs, capon, Cornish hen, pheasant | Pork | Lamb | Turkey | Beef |
| | | Shrimp, lobster, crab | Duck | Halibut, sole, turbot, flounder | Salmon, trout |
| | Tuna | | Scallops, clams, oysters | | |
| Vegetables | Lettuce | Carrot, celery, parsley, parsnip | White potato, tomato, eggplant | Yams | Cabbage, broccoli, Brussels sprouts, cauliflower, radish |
| | Onion, garlic, chives, leek, asparagus | | Spinach, beets | Legumes (peas, green beans, soy beans, lima beans) | Corn |
| | Artichoke | | Green pepper | Cucumber, squash, pumpkin, zucchini | |

**CHART 2. Five-Day Rotation Diet *(continued)***

| *Type of Food* | *Day 1* | *Day 2* | *Day 3* | *Day 4* | *Day 5* |
|---|---|---|---|---|---|
| Fruit | Apple, pear, quince<br>Papaya<br>Rhubarb<br>Figs, breadfruit | Citrus (orange, lime, lemon, grapefruit, tangerine, kumquat)<br>Banana, plantain, mango | Berries (raspberries, strawberries, blackberries)<br>Pineapple<br>Avocado | Cantaloupe, watermelon<br>Grapes, raisins<br>Coconut, dates<br>Blueberries, cranberries | Apricot, peach, plum, prune<br>Nectarine, cherries |
| Starch | Wheat, rye<br>Buckwheat | Arrowroot<br>Barley | Oats<br>Tapioca | Rice, rice flour<br>Soy flour | Cornstarch, cornmeal |
| Beverages | Apple juice<br>Mate tea<br>Papaya juice | Orange or grapefruit juice<br>Lemonade (sweetened with honey) | Tomato juice<br>Unsweetened pineapple juice<br>Sassafras tea | Unsweetened grape juice<br>Tea | Milk<br>Pure cocoa<br>Coffee |

| | | | | | |
|---|---|---|---|---|---|
| Nuts, seeds | Pecans, walnuts<br>Sunflower seeds | Cashews, pistachios<br>Sesame seeds | Brazil nuts<br>Macadamia nuts | Peanuts<br>Filberts<br>Melon seeds | Almonds |
| Oils | Sunflower oil<br>Walnut oil | Sesame oil<br>Olive oil<br>Cottonseed oil | Safflower oil, safflower oil margarine<br>Avocado oil | Peanut oil<br>Soy oil, soy margarine | Uncolored butter<br>Corn oil, corn oil margarine |
| Sweeteners | Cane sugar<br>Molasses | Honey<br>Barley malt syrup | Beet sugar | Saccharin<br>Date sugar | Maple syrup |
| Miscellaneous | Baker's yeast<br>Cider vinegar<br>Mushrooms | Allspice, cloves<br>Dill, cumin, caraway, coriander, fennel<br>Olives | Cinnamon, bayleaf, basil, sassafras, oregano, thyme, rosemary, peppermint, spearmint<br>Nutmeg, mace | Carob<br>Egg-replacer<br>Cream of tartar | Chocolate<br>Pure vanilla extract |

**CHART 3. Limited Four-Day Rotation Diet**

| Meal | Day 1 | Day 2 | Day 3 | Day 4 |
|---|---|---|---|---|
| Breakfast | Lamb | Almonds | Turkey | Cashews |
| Lunch | Pineapple | Grapes | Rice | Asparagus |
| Dinner | Carrots | Flounder | Shrimp | Bananas |
| Snack | Pecans | Cantaloupe | Pears | Grapefruit |

## KEEPING AWAY FROM CHEMICALS

What follows are some tips for reducing your exposure to chemicals without sacrificing cleanliness, comfort, or attractive surroundings. The extent *you* have to go to, to control *your* chemical sensitivities, is an individual matter. You may not need to carry out every avoidance measure to stay well. Still, it's never a bad idea to eliminate or replace unnecessary, possibly toxic products with safer ones. Remember: If you can smell a chemical that means it's entering your bloodstream. If you wouldn't eat that chemical, think twice before inhaling it or applying it to your skin! Unfortunately, even some of the suggested substitutions may bother some chemically sensitive people, so keep an eye open for reactions.

### Cleaning Chemicals

1. Throw away all bottles, boxes, and cans of the cleaning chemicals that cause your symptoms. Once they're open it's impossible to seal them tightly enough to keep them from polluting the air.
2. Avoid all aerosols.
3. Steer clear of products that warn they must be used only in a well-ventilated room.

4. Stay away from products containing chlorine, ammonia, petroleum, or offensive fragrances.
5. Use the following products and suggestions to replace any cleaning chemicals that make you sick.
   a. *Bathroom and kitchen cleansers*
      —Shaklee and Amway cleaning products. Shaklee's Basic H is often well tolerated and can be used for many chores.
      —Rokeach kosher soap (made from coconut oil).
      —Bon Ami, Arm & Hammer washing soda, Ivory, pure Castile soap.
      —Trisodium phosphate or oakite (poisonous, so use carefully).
      —Borax powder or baking soda, used as you would a powdered cleanser.
      —Vinegar, to cut soap film from tiles and to retard mold growth.
      —One-half bottle of cola substitutes, for toilet-bowl cleaner.
      —One-fourth cup of borax, for toilet-bowl cleaner (pour it into the toilet bowl, swirl with a toilet-bowl brush, and let stand 30 minutes before flushing).
   b. *Disinfectant*
      —Use borax, Zephiran (obtain from pharmacy), vinegar, and Impregnon for killing molds.
   c. *Brass cleanser*
      —Mix equal parts of salt and flour. Add vinegar to make a paste. Spread thick layer over brass. Let dry. Rinse and wipe off residue.
   d. *Oven cleaner*
      —Pour salt on a spill immediately. Wipe up with a damp sponge as soon as oven has cooled.
      —Use washing soda and plain steel wool.
      —Try Arm & Hammer oven cleaner.

e. *Silver polish*
 —Line bottom of a large pan with aluminum foil. Add 3 tablespoons baking powder to 1 quart water. Heat water in pan until almost boiling. Dip silver into water, making sure silver touches the foil. Immerse until tarnish disappears. Rinse. Dry and polish.
 —Apply toothpaste with a soft towel. Rinse well. Polish.

f. *Glass cleaner*
 —Add 1 tablespoon vinegar to 1 quart water. Pour into a pump spray bottle.

g. *Carpet cleaner*
 —Combine 2 cups cornmeal and 1 cup borax. Sprinkle over rug. Leave an hour. Vacuum thoroughly.
 —Sprinkle baking soda on carpet. Vacuum thoroughly.

h. *Dishwashing detergent*
 —Try Electra Sol (it's unscented).
 —Add 2 tablespoons vinegar to load of dishes to remove scum and detergents.
 —See if you can tolerate Palmolive dishwashing liquid, diluted with water. Use for washing dishes and pans by hand.

i. *Floor wax*
 —Try 1 capful baby oil (if tolerated) with tolerated detergent and water. Apply with a sponge, rinse, and polish with a soft cloth.

j. *Furniture polish*
 —Apply a thin layer of mayonnaise to a natural wood surface. Let stand 15 minutes. Then remove excess and polish with a soft cloth. Before trying this, however, spot-test the mayonnaise in a small, inconspicuous spot to make sure it won't damage your furniture.

—Use 100% pure lemon oil or raw linseed oil as you would furniture polish on natural wood surfaces. But spot-test for safety first.

k. *Laundry detergent and fabric softener*

—Put 1 cup vinegar in the final rinse cycle instead of fabric softener.

—If you react to a detergent, try a double rinse cycle. Add 1 cup vinegar to the rinse cycle.

—Substitute 1 cup borax with tolerated soap for bleach.

l. *Room deodorizer*

—Place a few drops of wintergreen oil on a cotton ball and put it somewhere out of sight in each room.

m. *Spot remover*

—Use 2 parts water to 1 part rubbing alcohol (if tolerated) in a well-ventilated room. Apply to spot and rub well until spot disappears. Then wash as usual.

**Cosmetics, Perfumes, and Other Personal Care Products**

1. Use as few cosmetic products as possible. Avoid perfumes and scented products.
2. Always read the list of ingredients. Try to pinpoint which ingredients cause symptoms.
3. Before using any new product, apply a small amount on the inside of your forearm and leave it on for 24 hours. If you have any adverse reaction at all, don't use the product.
4. Be aware that you can suddenly become sensitive to a cosmetic you've been using for years. The manufacturer may also change one of the ingredients.
5. If you do suspect a cosmetic allergy, wash the area well with bland soap. Stop using all cosmetics until the allergic reaction subsides. Then begin to experi-

ment using one cosmetic at a time, for one week each.

6. Try the following specific suggestions and replacements:
   a. *Deodorants*
      —Choose unscented, nonaerosol deodorants.
      —Add 2 tablespoons alum to 1 pint warm water. Dab on underarms with cotton ball.
      —Lightly dust underarms with baking soda.
   b. *Shaving*
      —Use an electric razor to avoid shaving cream. Skip aftershave lotion.
   c. *Sanitary products*
      —Use unscented tampons or sanitary napkins made of natural fibers.
   d. *Hair care products*
      —For dry hair, apply ½ cup mayonnaise to dry, unwashed hair. Cover with a towel. After 15 minutes, rinse. Then shampoo thoroughly.
      —For a dry shampoo, if you're in a hurry, mix together 1 tablespoon salt and ½ cup cornmeal. Sprinkle over oily hair. Then brush thoroughly to remove dirt.
      —Try out such commercial shampoos as Johnson's Baby Shampoo, Amino Pon, Almay, and Castile shampoo, which may be tolerated. Avoid products containing formaldehyde or offensive fragrances.
      —Use natural hair dyes like henna.
      —For a hair setting lotion, dissolve 1 teaspoon sugar or gelatin in 1 cup water. Pour into pump spray bottle. Apply to wet hair and comb through.
   e. *Lip balm*
      —Melt equal parts of beeswax and safflower oil in a small pan over low heat. Remove from

stove. Whip quickly with a fork until mixture thickens. Store at room temperature.

f. *Toothpaste*
   —See if you can tolerate a natural toothpaste brand.
   —As a substitute, mix 2 tablespoons salt with ¾ cup baking soda in blender until finely ground. Add 2 teaspoons of pure mint extract (if tolerated). Blend well. Add just enough water to moisten into a paste. Store in covered glass jar.

g. *Mouthwash*
   —Add ½ teaspoon pure mint extract to 8 ounces of water.

**Drugs**

1. Avoid taking drugs if at all possible. Drugs consumed in the greatest quantity and taken most frequently are the ones most likely to cause problems. Don't demand prescriptions from your doctor, but don't refuse medication if it's really needed.
2. Be sure your doctor knows all the drugs you're taking—over-the-counter medications, vitamins, minerals, and prescriptions from any other doctors. Make a list.
3. Be wary of over-the-counter medications. Do you absolutely need them? Do they really help? (Consult Joe Graedon's books, listed in Appendix F.)
4. When you do take a prescription drug, be sure you know the name of the drug. Take the medication exactly as your doctor orders.
5. If you're sensitive to artificial colorings, ask your doctor if there is an uncolored tablet that will do just as well. Colored coatings can be washed off in many cases, but ask your pharmacist or doctor first.

Colored capsules can be emptied into clear gelatin ones supplied by your pharmacist.

6. If you are sensitive to materials used as fillers, check with your doctor, pharmacist, or the manufacturer to see if the offending material is used in that drug.

**Fabrics**

1. If you're sensitive to synthetic fibers, try 100% pure cotton, untreated wool, or silk.
2. If a fabric feels or smells offensive, don't buy it.
3. Test fabrics with a formaldehyde test kit (see Appendix B).
4. Check out this clue as to whether a fabric has been finished with chemicals: Drop a bubble of water on the fabric in an inconspicuous spot. If the bubble remains without soaking in, the fabric has probably been treated.
5. Look for all-cotton sheets, pads, and blankets. Older relatives or friends may have some all-cotton sheets they aren't using anymore. All-wool blankets may be tolerated. Make quilts from all-cotton batting and all-cotton fabrics.
6. Cover synthetic mattresses with all-cotton quilts or blankets. Don't use plastics.
7. Avoid carpeting. Use all-cotton scatter rugs or untreated all-wool rugs.

**Formaldehyde**

1. Get a formaldehyde test kit to check the formaldehyde levels in both your indoor air and any product you're considering buying (see Appendix B). Your local or state board of health may test samples of your indoor air for formaldehyde if requested by your doctor. In some states this service is free.

2. To neutralize formaldehyde in the air, put 1 tablespoon ammonia in a bucket of water in each room. Keep your house closed for several hours. Then, air the house well upon your return. Repeat this procedure every few months, or as needed. What happens is that the ammonia unites with the formaldehyde to form a harmless chemical.
3. Steer clear of particle board shelves, furniture, or cabinets. Or seal them well with paint or shellac. But keep them out of the house until the paint or shellac fumes dissipate completely.
4. Avoid carpeting, if possible. Choose attractive, tolerated flooring (brick, hardwood, stone, terrazzo, cement, ceramic tiles, and some vinyl). Choose adhesives carefully.
5. If your carpet store is cooperative, ask them to air out new carpeting in their warehouse for you.
6. Choose furniture carefully. Formica and hard plastics may be tolerated. If possible, use natural fabrics for slipcovers and upholstery.
7. Always prewash new fabrics and clothes well before you use them.
8. Stay away from homes with urea-formaldehyde foam insulation. Yellow fiberglass wrapped in aluminum is the best-tolerated insulation.
9. Avoid all cosmetics and personal care products that contain formaldehyde or Formalin.

### Newsprint, Inks, and Office Supplies

1. Use mechanical lead pencils instead of regular wooden ones.
2. Avoid felt-tip pens. Test if you tolerate metal pens better than plastic ones.
3. Steer clear of scented paper and pens with scented inks.

4. Try a typewriter with a ribbon cartridge instead of a ribbon spool. Also see if a second-hand typewriter is less offensive, as it should have aired out.
5. Avoid using correction fluid for typing errors; type-over correction paper is preferred.
6. Choose milk-based glues over those with toxic fumes.
7. Buy self-sticking envelopes to avoid licking them.
8. If you are in charge of buying a new copying machine, check various brands, as some are less offensive than others.
9. Dry hardcover books in oven at 200° for an hour to reduce odor.
10. Cover pages of any book to be read with cellophane.
11. Avoid blown-in cellulosic home insulation, which is made from ground-up newspapers plus fire-retardant chemicals.

**Paints**

1. Paint only in the spring or summer and leave the windows open as much as possible.
2. Don't use oil-based paints.
3. Try Dupont Lucite (without Teflon or Hexylate), which may be tolerated. Add baking soda a little at a time, stirring well until bubbles stop. Casein-type paints may also be tolerated.
4. Stick as much as possible to white and off-white colors, as they may be tolerated better than tinted paints.
5. To help neutralize the odor, add 2 teaspoons vanilla extract per 1 quart paint. Or try one large onion cut in half in a large pan of cold water. You may also use an electronic air cleaner with a charcoal filter to absorb paint odors.

**Pesticides**

1. Remove all containers of pesticides, mothballs, and fly strips from the house.
2. Use fly swatters, mousetraps, and natural chemicals to kill pests. Or use Ultra-Sonic Pest Control, which emits ultrahigh-intensity sound waves that drive all types of pests away (see Appendix B). Consult Natalie Golos' and Frances Golbitz's *Coping with Your Allergies* for natural pest control suggestions (see Appendix F).
3. To keep mosquitoes from biting you outdoors, try 100 milligrams of thiamine (vitamin $B_1$), taken orally, before an exposure.
4. Stay indoors when your neighborhood is sprayed for mosquitoes or your neighbors' lawns are fertilized.

**Petroleum Products and Gas Fumes**

1. If you have a gas stove, disconnect it and seal off the gas pipes to see if your symptoms improve. If yes, replace the gas stove with an electric one. Corningware electric stoves with no wire burners are well tolerated.
2. If you have a gas furnace, ask your gas company to check it for small leaks. Better yet, replace it with an electric one. Or relocate the gas furnace in a separate enclosure outside the house. Although electrical baseboard heating is dust- and chemical-free, it is the most expensive alternative.
3. Replace any gas or kerosene heaters with electric ones.
4. Substitute electric appliances for gas water heaters and dryers.
5. Keep all drains in the basement full of water to prevent sewer gas from backing up into the house.
6. If your garage is connected to your house or,

worse yet, located underneath the house, try parking the car outside. Clean up all grease and oil spills by spreading kitty litter or sand over the spots. Allow the particles to absorb the petroleum products. Then sweep up and discard.

7. Have your car's exhaust system checked carefully for leaks.
8. In traffic, keep your windows shut and don't drive too close to the vehicle in front of you. Leave early or late to avoid traffic jams. Take an alternative route that is less congested. Buy an electronic air filter for your car.
9. Use an electric lawn mower instead of a gasoline-powered one.
10. Avoid soft, smelly plastics. Hard plastics like Formica can usually be tolerated.
11. Instead of a plastic shower curtain, use an all-cotton sheet. Or hang the plastic curtain outside until it is thoroughly aired out.
12. Store food in stainless steel or glass containers. Use cellophane food bags instead of plastic. When using foil, wrap food with the shiny side next to the food, as the dull side is coated with plastic. Use Corningware, Pyrex, stainless steel, or iron cooking utensils, not Teflon.

**Phenol**

1. Don't use cleaning products containing phenol or carbolic acid.
2. If possible, avoid medical injections containing phenol.
3. Keep away from throat lozenges or sprays, cough drops, and mouthwashes that contain phenol.

**Pine**

1. Steer clear of pine-scented products such as some cosmetics, deodorizers, cleansers, and soaps.

2. Don't use pine, spruce, cedar, or redwood paneling.
3. Avoid turpentine.
4. Buy an artificial Christmas tree. But check its odor before purchasing it to see if you can tolerate it.

**Tobacco**

1. If you're a smoker, quit! (Much easier said than done.)
2. If you have a smoker in the house, ask him or her to smoke outside. If this is impossible, confine any smoking to one, closed-up room with an electronic air filter.
3. Request seating in no-smoking sections of airplanes and restaurants.

**Water**

1. Boil water for 10 minutes to remove chlorine.
2. Add a pinch of ascorbic acid (vitamin C) crystals to a glass of water to neutralize the chlorine for drinking.
3. Add a few sodium thiosulfate crystals to bath water to neutralize chlorine. This is *not* for drinking.
4. Locate an uncontaminated local spring or well. Store water in glass jugs.
5. Buy bottled spring water in glass jugs, although bottled water is expensive long-term.
6. Distill or filter your own water. Try to rent a distillation or filtration unit before purchasing it to see if you can tolerate the water (see Appendix B).

# 7

# Doctors' Procedures for Diagnosing and Treating *Your* Allergies

It's a good idea to have your suspected sensitivities checked by a nontraditional allergist. What can you expect from a visit? First, the doctor will take a detailed family and personal medical history, looking for clues that suggest allergies and possible allergens. Here's where your answers to the questions in Chapter 3 and your Exposure Diary (Chapter 5) may be particularly helpful. The doctor will also conduct a physical exam, searching for signs of allergy, nutritional deficiencies, or other abnormalities. Let's look at some of the specific allergy tests you may encounter.

## BLOOD TESTS

Several blood tests are available that may help your doctor decide if your problems are allergy-related and just what they might be. The possibilities include:

1. *Complete Blood Count:* If the eosinophils (a type of white blood cell) are elevated above 3% in your white blood count, allergy may be present.
2. *IgE Blood Test:* This test measures the total immunoglobulin E, an antibody associated with most allergies. A high IgE indicates that allergy may be present. But a low IgE doesn't necessarily mean that allergies aren't present.
3. *RAST (Radio-Allergo-Sorbant Test):* In this test the focus in on the amount of immunoglobulin E present for specific allergens such as molds, dust, pollens, stinging insects, and some foods (including milk, egg, wheat, and fish). Your doctor specifies which allergens are tested for (the more allergens tested for, the more expensive the RAST is). If the RAST indicates a high level of IgE antibodies for a particular allergen, that's a good indication you are sensitive to it. Again, however, a low level of IgE antibodies does not necessarily rule out that substance as a cause of your symptoms. Not all allergies are IgE-mediated.
4. *Cytoxic Blood Test.* This test identifies particular food allergies and some chemical and drug allergies. All the foods to be tested for should be eaten a few days before the test. Live white blood cells are mixed with each allergen extract to be tested. If the white blood cells are damaged or destroyed by a food extract, you are probably sensitive to that food. The test is not 100% accurate, but it may be helpful in identifying problem foods. Again, however, the more allergens tested for, the more expensive the test. Another problem is that this test is only reliable if performed by highly trained lab personnel. In addition, the blood tested must be fresh, so the patient must visit the lab in person. The test is not available in every city.

## ■ INHALANT ALLERGY TESTING AND TREATMENT

Traditional allergists use *scratch tests* to check inhalant allergies. Suspected individual antigens are dropped on the skin and then slightly scratched into the surface. Or the extract may be injected into the skin. The doctor waits to see if any swelling or redness occurs at each site, indicating a positive reaction. Then, desensitizing injections of small amounts of the offending allergens may be given, with the dosage gradually increased. These injections are most effective against ragweed, cats, stinging insects, and tree pollens; for some, they may be less effective against house dust and molds. Dosage must be carefully monitored. Too little extract may be ineffective, while an overdose can cause anaphylactic shock.

Other allergists use the *titration method* for inhalant testing and treatment. Weak extracts of the suspected substances are injected under the skin in a vertical row, down the upper arm. After ten minutes each injection site is measured to see if the wheal has increased in size, indicating the patient is sensitive to that allergen. When such a positive reaction is found, a weaker dose is then injected to determine a dilution of the extract that can be tolerated. On the other hand, if the initial reaction is negative, a stronger dilution is used to determine where the tolerance point is.

The titration system may allow the doctor to start treatment with stronger doses, so symptoms are alleviated sooner. Once the tolerated doses are determined, the various allergens are mixed together to make the patient's treatment dose. This dose is usually given once a week by injection in the doctor's office, or sometimes every few days using sublingual (under the tongue) drops. The idea is to gradually increase the dose so that the patient's body increases its tolerance for the various allergens but doesn't react to the allergy shots themselves. Along with the allergy shots, of course, patients should try to reduce their exposure to allergens.

## ■ PROVOCATIVE TESTING AND NEUTRALIZATION FOR FOODS AND CHEMICALS

Unfortunately, scratch tests are not very reliable for foods. Problem foods may cause no skin reactions or harmless foods may appear positive. If your doctor suspects food and chemical allergies, he or she may ask you to carry out elimination diets and chemical sniff tests at home (see Chapter 5). Another possibility is a rotation diet (see Chapter 6). Or your doctor may decide to conduct provocative food and chemical tests.

Provocative testing and neutralization for foods and chemicals not only allow both patient and doctor to see which substances cause symptoms, but can also be used as a form of treatment to prevent or "turn off" symptoms. Your doctor may do either intradermal (under the skin) or sublingual provocative testing, working with various dilutions, one at a time.

Suppose corn is the prime suspect in your case. A small amount of corn extract is either injected under your skin or dropped under your tongue. Both your physical and mental reactions are carefully noted. With intradermal testing, your skin reaction is also measured. Then, ten minutes later, another dilution of the corn extract is administered. Again, your reactions are recorded. This process is repeated until your doctor is sure no symptoms have been provoked (indicating you are not sensitive to corn), or a dose is reached that neutralizes any reaction. This neutral point indicates the *treatment* dose. You would take this dose every day, under your tongue, at home—or several times a week by injection. This neutralizing dose allows you to eat one serving of corn each day without developing symptoms (although less frequent servings are preferred). If you eat too much corn, you'll experience symptoms again.

Let's look at an example of a patient being tested intradermally for corn. Every time "Paul" eats corn he gets a bad headache. At 10:00 A.M. a dilution of corn extract at 1 to 500 parts is injected under his skin and is measured immediately. Ten minutes later, the wheal is measured again, its characteristics described, and any symptoms noted. The record of Paul's corn test is shown in Chart 4.

So Paul's treatment dose for corn is 1 part corn extract to 62,500 parts of water. This dose will allow him to eat a serving of corn once every few days without getting a headache or any other symptoms.

Provocative testing for inhalants and chemicals works the same way. Common chemicals tested are ethanol (which helps protect the patient while exposed to petroleum products), phenol, formaldehyde, chlorine, tobacco smoke, perfume, newsprint, artificial colorings, and preservatives. Secretaries sensitive to carbon paper have been tested and treated sublingually, using an extract made from carbon paper. Teachers allergic to chalk and mimeograph paper have also been successfully treated. Remember, however, that these neutralizing chemical doses don't provide relief for *constant* exposures.

If you have inhalant allergies but can't tolerate traditional inhalant-extract injections, provocative testing and treatment for phenol—a preservative used in the inhalant extract—may bring relief. If you still can't tolerate traditional inhalant-extract therapy, provocative tests can be used for each offending inhalant. You

**CHART 4. Sample Results of Provocative Corn Test**

| *Time* | *Corn Dose* | *Wheal Size Right After Injection* | *Wheal Size and Type 10 Minutes Later* | *Symptoms* |
|---|---|---|---|---|
| 10:00 | 1:500 | 7 × 7 millimeters (mm) | 9 × 9 mm (hard, raised—a positive wheal) | Slight headache |
| 10:10 | 1:2500 | 7 × 7 mm | 9 × 9 mm (hard, raised—a positive wheal) | Headache worse, dark circles under eyes, runny nose, sneezing |
| 10:20 | 1:12500 | 7 × 7 mm | 7 × 7 mm (soft—a negative wheal) | Headache a little better, nose still running, circles still dark |
| 10:30 | 1:62500 | 7 × 7 mm | 7 × 7 mm (soft—a negative wheal) | Headache gone, nose clear, dark circles better |
| 10:40 | No dose | | | Still feels good, dark circles gone |

would then be treated with neutralizing doses instead of gradually increasing doses.

The success of provocative testing depends on the skill and experience of the person doing the testing. Because each test may require from 30 minutes to several hours to attain a neutralizing dose, the process is time-consuming and expensive. Avoidance is still the preferred "treatment," but when that is impossible, provocative testing and neutralization treatment can be very effective.

It's true that traditional allergists dismiss provocative testing as so much subjective hocus-pocus. Clinical ecologists and other doctors who use this method freely admit they don't know yet why provocative testing works. But they have found it very effective. Their patients are usually amazed at how their symptoms can be turned on and off with different dilutions of the extraction. One minute they feel fine, the next they feel wretched. When the neutralizing dose is given, they feel fine again.

## ■ RELIEF FOR BAD REACTIONS

Most clinical ecologists believe that the least medication prescribed for any patient (particularly the chemically sensitive) is best. As alternatives, they may suggest that you try one or more of the following innocuous remedies when you have a bad reaction.

1. Exercise to increase the oxygen supply and to help rid the body of excess water. In some cases, breathing oxygen (a prescription) is very helpful.
2. Suck on an ice cube; it sometimes eases symptoms.
3. Retire to the one room in your house (your

"oasis") that you have made as allergy-free as possible.

4. Do relaxation exercises (see Chapter 13).
5. Take Alka-Seltzer Gold, an aspirin-free medication that often brings dramatic relief of allergy symptoms. It should be taken with at least 8 ounces of water, preferably 16 ounces. Because of its high sodium content, however, use should be limited to once a day or as recommended by your doctor. Patient on salt-restricted diets should avoid it.
6. Prepare your own alkaline salts remedy: Mix together 2 parts baking soda (sodium bicarbonate) with 1 part potassium bicarbonate. Place 1 heaping teaspoon of this mixture in 16 ounces of water. Again, caution is needed as this remedy is high in sodium.
7. Use plain milk of magnesia, as directed on the label, to empty the system of foods that are causing a reaction.
8. Try vitamin-C tablets or powder, 500 to 1000 milligrams every hour or so, until symptoms subside. Gas or diarrhea is a sign that you're taking too much vitamin C. Slightly reduce your dose until the gas or diarrhea subsides. Nutricology makes a special vitamin-C powder that contains calcium, magnesium, and potassium (see Appendix B). It is similar to Alka-Seltzer Gold but contains vitamin C and no sodium. The powder comes in two forms: One is made from corn; the other is corn-free and derived from sago palm.
9. See if extra pantothenic acid (vitamin $B_5$), in doses of 500 to 1000 milligrams, reduces symptoms.
10. Try selenium, which may help reduce reactions to chemicals. Nutricology puts out an allergy formula containing selenium for this purpose (see Appendix B).

Your doctor may suggest an antihistamine tablet. Optimine, Tavist, and Periactin are dye-free, prescription antihistamines. Benadryl comes in a slightly colored capsule, but the contents can be emptied into a clear gelatin capsule. Common side effects are drowsiness, which may subside after taking antihistamines awhile. Or another type of antihistamine may be better tolerated.

## ENVIRONMENTAL HOSPITAL UNITS

If you're experiencing very severe symptoms that haven't responded to any form of treatment, your doctor may consider hospitalizing you in a special environmental care unit. Unfortunately, because there are only a few units in the United States (see Appendix B), there is often a long waiting list for admission. And, like all hospital care, these units are expensive; they can cost thousands of dollars for several weeks of care. Not all insurance companies will pay for this specialized care, so check in advance if you are considering entering an ecological unit.

An ecological unit provides a clean, uncontaminated environment. The air is filtered to keep out all dust, molds, pollens, and chemicals. The unit itself is isolated from the odors of the rest of the hospital. The water comes from very deep wells or is carefully filtered. Only well-tolerated cleaning chemicals are used. Rooms and furniture are decorated and chosen with care. Beds have cotton sheets and mattresses. Hospital personnel, often allergy victims themselves, wear all-cotton clothes and avoid using scented products. Patients, too, wear all-natural fibers (cotton, wool, linen, or silk); they are not allowed to wear or bring anything into the unit that might bother someone else. Flowers, tobacco, cosmetics, perfumes, plastics, scented soaps, deodorants, toothpaste, freshly printed material, and outside food—all are strictly forbidden.

What would it be like for you in such a unit? When you first enter, you fast for four to six days on nothing but spring water. As much medication as possible is stopped. Laxatives are given to thoroughly clean out your system. During the first few days you may experience a severe withdrawal reaction and your symptoms may get worse. After four or five days, however, you may well feel better than you have in years.

The next step, after the fast, is to try different bottled and chlorinated waters to see which ones you tolerate best. Then, additive-free foods are reintroduced, one at a time, and any reaction noted. Only a few foods are tested each day. You are also tested for various inhalants by inhaling them in powder form, one at a time, while symptoms are carefully monitored. If severe symptoms occur, provocative testing is done to find a neutralizing dose that turns off the symptoms and can be used for protection.

Sniff tests are also carried out for various chemicals, such as gas fumes, newsprint, and tobacco. Neutralizing doses are found if possible. But primarily you are taught how to avoid these chemicals and how to change your home and work environments to accommodate your sensitivities.

Tests for too much or too little hydrochloric acid in the stomach may be run, since either extreme can be a factor in food allergy. In addition, you may be asked to eat offending foods with pancreatic enzymes to see if this enables you to tolerate them. For some patients, the enzymes are quite helpful; for others, they seem to speed up the reaction.

Finally, you will try eating foods that you can tolerate in a chemical-free form. But this time you will eat commercial foods, with chemical additives and contaminants. It may be that you can tolerate only organically grown foods. On your last day in the unit, you'll wear your normal street clothes and personal care products to see if these bother you.

Before returning home, you are advised to arrange for one room in your home to be made into an "oasis," a place that is as close to the hospital environment as possible so that when you experience symptoms you can go there to recuperate. Once you've resumed a normal routine at home, you can return to work. Obviously, any offending substances there should be noted.

One of the goals of these hospital units is patient education. As a patient, you attend seminars and group discussions led by the doctors and nurses, visit with other patients, and read as much as possible so that you will be well-equipped to deal with your individual problems when you go home. Some of the necessary changes in lifestyle may be quite expensive, frustrating, and time-consuming. But they may be literally lifesaving for some sensitive people.

# SECTION THREE

# Correcting Factors That Make You Susceptible to Allergies

# 8

# Heredity and Infant Feeding—an Ounce of Prevention

Why are some people allergy-prone and others not? Are there underlying biochemical factors that promote allergies? Can certain factors make allergies worse? These questions go beyond the allergens themselves. The issue is why only some people react adversely and others do not. Certainly we still have a lot to learn about which factors promote allergies. And even in what we do know, much remains controversial.

It's unlikely that we'll find a simple answer to the question of why a particular person is afflicted with allergies. There is probably a combination of reasons. Suppose a young woman with a strong family history of allergies has eaten a nutritionally deficient diet for years. Her teeth have decayed so her mouth is full of silver-mercury fillings. Her marriage is stormy and stressful. She's on birth control pills. She's run down and at some point gets the flu. Her doctor gives her antibiotics. A chronic yeast infection sets in. Gradually this woman develops a host of physical and mental symptoms, caused by multiple allergies. It's no surprise. A number of precipitating factors can be identified in the description of her life. Controlling them as much as possible, plus avoiding her allergens, may lead to dramatic improvement or the disappearance of her allergy symptoms. The same might be true for you.

Allergies tend to run in families. If you are allergic, you probably have more allergic relatives than a nonallergic person does. Both genetic and family environmental factors may be contributing to your allergy-proneness. Studies that were looking only for traditionally recognized allergy symptoms found that two allergic parents had a 75% chance of having an allergic child. If only one parent was allergic, the chance of having an allergic child dropped to 50%.[1]

In reviewing a family history, nontraditional allergists include a much broader range of symptoms than the traditionally recognized ones. Keeping in mind that my own family is unusually allergic, let's look at an abbreviated family medical history for one of my sons:

1. *Mother*
   —Food allergies and grass pollen allergies as a child.
   —Sugar addiction.
   —Fatigue, achiness, joint pain, depression, frequent "bugs," and gallbladder attacks as an adult caused by sensitivities to multiple foods, inhalants, and chemicals.
   —Sensitivity to sulfa, severe reactions (shock) to stinging insects, severe reactions to poison ivy.
2. *Maternal Grandmother*
   —Food allergies as a child and adult causing joint pain and stiffness, low blood sugar, headaches,

sinus troubles, gallbladder attacks, and possibly high blood pressure.

3. *Maternal Uncle (mother's only sibling)*
   —Asthma, hay fever, colitis, headaches, and gallbladder disorder.
4. *Father*
   —Tonsillitis as a child.
   —Cola addiction.
   —Puffiness, sinus difficulties, runny nose, fatigue, indigestion, hiatal hernia, aching muscles, and gallbladder trouble as an adult due to sensitivities to inhalants, foods, and chemicals.
   —Bad reactions to stinging insects and poison ivy.
5. *Paternal Aunt (father's only sibling)*
   —Asthma as a child.
6. *Brother*
   —Hyperactivity, leg aches, headaches, runny nose, and eczema due to multiple inhalant, food, and chemical allergies.

Of course, there's nothing you can do to change your genes. But you *can* help future family members, if there is a hereditary tendency to allergies, by controlling other contributing factors as much as possible.

## PRENATAL CARE

"An ounce of prevention is worth a pound of cure" goes the old saying. And allergic parents planning a baby would do well to follow this advice. It's much easier to be cautious before and after birth than it is to control a child's or adult's multiple allergies.

There are no guarantees, but doctors who work with allergic families believe that the severity of a baby's future allergic problems can be significantly reduced by good prenatal care.[2] And whether allergies are involved or not, doctors believe that every child can benefit from proper nutrition, both prenatally and during the early years.

Ideally, both the mother and the father will have been practicing good nutrition for years before conception. But it's never too late to start. Once the mother is pregnant, she needs to watch her diet closely. What she eats during pregnancy will affect the emotional, mental, and physical development of her child. She needs to keep herself in optimal condition. If the mother suffers from allergies, the stress of pregnancy may make them worse.

Eating a well-balanced diet; avoiding lots of sugar, caffeine, salt, and additives; taking vitamin and mineral supplements as prescribed by her doctor (preferably unflavored and uncolored); and steering clear of foods she knows she's sensitive to—all this will help the expectant mother feel better and benefit her unborn child. If allergies run in the family, some doctors advise staying away from or cutting down on such highly allergenic foods as milk and eggs. They also recommend that the mother vary her diet as much as possible and avoid eating large quantities of any one food. Some women don't normally drink much milk because they dislike it or know it doesn't make them feel good. But as soon as they become pregnant, they think they need to drink a lot. Consequently, they may feel worse, and they may help to sensitize their children to milk. After all, cows don't drink milk to produce healthy calves, nor do they need to drink milk in order to nurse them! The pregnant mother just needs to be sure she is getting the protein, calcium, and vitamins that milk would supply.

If possible, the pregnant mother should avoid stress. Stress before, during, or after birth may increase the likelihood of future allergies. Pregnant women should also avoid all unnecessary medications unless carefully prescribed by a doctor. Recent evidence shows that many drugs do cross the placenta and enter the baby's bloodstream. Caution and discretion, by both mother and doctor, are recommended. Similarly, smoking and coffee and alcohol consumption should be decreased, or given up. So should chemical exposures.

## ■ FEEDING YOUR INFANT

Both traditional and nontraditional allergists, as well as many pediatricians, recognize that inadequate infant feeding practices can promote allergies. Breast-fed babies are much less likely to develop allergies than formula-fed babies. The lining of the infant's intestines is thought to be quite permeable to food proteins. Although mother's milk proteins are tolerated, cow's milk proteins may be allergenic. Go to the store and read the labels on the baby formulas. They contain cow's milk, sugar, and corn. Early exposure to these foods makes them prime candidates for causing allergy. Even soy milk formulas contain sugar and corn. Breast-feeding is cheaper, more convenient, more nutritious, and more emotionally satisfying for both mother and child. There is one qualification: The practice of feeding sugar water to the newborn before the mother's milk comes in should be discouraged.

If at all possible, the new mother should plan to breast-feed for at least four to six months. But even a few weeks is beneficial. With more new mothers returning to work, breast-feeding becomes more difficult. Some mothers feel so strongly about the benefits of breast milk, compared with formulas, that they use a breast pump so that their milk can be given by bottle to the baby when they're not home. But this takes a lot of dedication, and it isn't possible for all new mothers. If you wean your baby from the breast before a year, consider using a milk substitute instead of cow's milk—especially if there's a family history of milk allergy.

While breast-feeding, continue to watch your diet closely—you are still eating for two. What you eat will affect your baby. If your baby develops colic or spits up frequently, you should keep a diet diary, recording what you eat and drink. See if there is any relationship between a change in your diet and your baby's reaction. A prime suspect is cow's milk, but eggs, chocolate, citrus, and wheat also commonly present problems. If the mother is sensitive to a food she eats, the baby may also react. But the baby may also react to a food the mother is not sensitive to. Think twice before switching a colicky, sickly baby off breast milk. The very babies who are fussy and irritable on breast milk often do even worse on formula.[3]

Vitamin drops may also be a problem for the colicky baby. Some babies are sensitive to the fillers, sugar, or artificial colorings and flavorings in these; others seem to be sensitive to the vitamin sources—for example, cod liver oil. To check if vitamin drops are a problem, stop them for five days and see if your baby's symptoms improve. Then, reintroduce the drops and note any reactions. Consult your doctor if a reaction occurs.

Early introduction of solid foods may lead to allergies, as the proteins in them are foreign to the baby's immune system. Many doctors believe that infants (particularly ones with allergic parents or siblings) should only be breast-fed for the first three to six months. Introduction of any solid foods should be postponed. The longer you wait, the better the chances your child won't become sensitive to the new foods. This may make you feel uneasy, and you may be criticized by relatives and friends who all started solids earlier. Your baby doesn't need these foods in the early months. If your baby has colic, it's likely that feeding solids won't ease the crying and may just sensitize the child. Try contacting a La Leche League in your area; you may find this group supportive and full of helpful information.

When you do start solids, you should begin with rice or oat cereals.[4] Mix these either with breast milk or water—not formula or cow's milk. Leave wheat until at least nine months of age.

Fruits may be started at four months or preferably six. But apples, peaches, citrus fruits, and berries should be withheld longer. Postpone raw fruit until 12 months (except bananas), citrus fruits until 18 months, and berries until 24 months. Bananas, pears, plums, and apricots are least likely to cause problems.

Vegetables may be introduced at four to six months, beginning with carrots. Beets, squash, asparagus, sweet potato, and white potato are likely to be tolerated well. Don't offer peas, beans, or spinach until your baby is a year old. Wait another six months before adding tomatoes, leaving corn until age two.

Between six and nine months, strained meats like lamb and veal, then pork and beef, can be started. Save liver and chicken until last. Don't introduce eggs until at least nine months and preferably a year. Then start with small amounts of hard-cooked egg yolk, adding a little hard-cooked egg white if the yolks are tolerated. Chocolate, nuts, and nut butters should be withheld until two to three years of age.

Here is a quick guide for when to introduce solids:

*0 to 6 months*
—Breast milk
*4 to 6 months*
—Rice and oat cereals
—Bananas; cooked pears, plums, and apricots

—Carrots, beets, squash, asparagus, sweet potato, and white potato

*6 to 9 months*

—Lamb and veal, then pork and beef, with chicken and liver last

—Apples and peaches

*9 to 12 months*

—Hard-cooked egg yolks; if egg yolks are tolerated, hard-cooked egg whites

—Wheat

*12 months (1 year)*

—Raw fruits (not citrus or berries)

—Peas, beans, and spinach

*18 months*

—Citrus fruits and juices

—Tomatoes

*24 months (2 years)*

—Berries

—Corn

*24 to 36 months (2 to 3 years)*

—Chocolate, nuts, and nut butters

Give your baby only a teaspoon of the new food at a time, doubling the amount each day until a full serving is reached. Don't introduce a new food more often than once every three days. Some doctors believe that allergic babies do better if they are not fed the same foods every day and each food is only used once in four or five days—a kind of rotation diet.

What symptoms should you watch for? Increased fussiness, wheezing, diarrhea, rashes, vomiting, "colds," and coughing may be signs of a food sensitivity. Of course, these problems may have other causes too. Keep a careful food diary, noting your baby's age, the foods given, and any reactions. Don't use food mixtures because you won't be able to pinpoint which ingredient causes the symptoms. And don't give any one food too often or in extra-large portions.

If you are tempted to speed up this schedule, listen to some advice from the Allergy Information Association of Canada:

> The baby doesn't need it. It is you that needs the variety. Fast feeding is beneficial to the baby food companies, not to your baby. Fast feeding is a symptom of our hurry, flurry world. Above all, remember that how you feed the baby in the first year will affect him all his life. He will be what he eats.[5]

Another question: Should you buy baby food or make your own? Either way, there are pros and cons. You'll have to decide what's best for you, your lifestyle, and your baby. Fortunately, baby food companies have made an effort to improve their products by removing salt, preservatives, and artificial colorings and flavorings, as well as reducing or eliminating sugar. But many products still contain sweeteners, so always read labels carefully. Keep away from mixtures such as mixed vegetables, cereals, dinners, and desserts. If you buy strained bananas, you may find other ingredients such as orange juice added, which you'll want to avoid introducing for awhile. Because teething biscuits and crackers all contain bleached flour, corn syrup, and sugar, they should be avoided. Juices may contain sugar or corn sweetener. Don't use a bottle of milk or juice as a pacifier at nap- or bedtime as the natural sugars will promote tooth decay.

Once your child is old enough to eat what the rest of the family is eating, be sure to keep his or her diet nutritious and free from sugary, nutritionally empty snacks. It'll help your child feel, look, and act better.

"Fingerfoods" such as raw carrots, celery, slices of fruit, cheese (if milk is tolerated), and bits of meat should be encouraged at the appropriate age. In general, children who start life on the best foods, and continue eating them in their early years, won't crave sweets and junk foods. They'll grow up demanding good, nutritious food.

## ■ ADDITIONAL ADVICE

Try to keep your baby's room as clean and free of allergens as possible. A room with washable items, few dust-catchers, and no rugs may help. One doctor found that installing an electronic air cleaner in his grandchild's house promptly brought an end to the child's colic. Your baby may be sensitive to synthetic fibers, disposable diapers, lotions, and soaps. Don't use room deodorizers, pesticide strips, or aerosol sprays. Smoking should not be allowed around the baby.

Keep in mind that allergic reactions in children are not limited to asthma, hay fever, and rashes. Stomachaches, headaches, leg pains, and dizziness often have an allergic origin. Behavior problems, including temper tantrums, hyperactivity, violence, fatigue, depression, and Dr. Jekyll–Mr. Hyde personality changes, may also be allergic reactions. The same goes for learning difficulties. Children with pale, washed-out complexions, who are always tired or overactive, and have dark, puffy circles under their eyes, should be checked for allergy.

Many traditional allergists won't test and treat a child under five, but clinical ecologists believe it's important to recognize and treat the allergic child as soon as possible. Small children (even babies) have been safely tested with provocative allergy techniques.

# 9

# Candida Albicans: A Beastly Yeast

The most exciting recent development in identifying what promotes allergy is the discovery that a yeast infection can weaken the body's immune system so much that the person becomes chronically ill. The yeast involved is Candida albicans. The form the chronic illness takes depends on the individual and his or her genetic weak links. Possible symptoms range from severe psychological problems, to multiple allergies, to other diseases with an immunological basis such as lupus, myasthenia gravis, rheumatoid arthritis, Crohn's disease, and multiple sclerosis.[1] Clearing the yeast infection with diet, anti-yeast drugs, and Candida extract injections often brings dramatic relief of symptoms.

But what is Candida albicans? Candida is a yeast organism living in everyone. Normally it inhabits the mouth, esophagus, intestines, vagina, and skin. As long as our immune system keeps it in balance, it doesn't cause problems. And, although minor infections were recognized, until recently few researchers considered it a common factor in serious health problems. Then, in 1961, allergist C. Orian Truss found that one of his patients, who suffered from runny nose, migraine headaches, depression, and a vaginal yeast infection, repeatedly experienced complete relief from all her symptoms when she received an injection of Candida extract. Several years later Dr. Truss tried this therapy with other patients and again achieved success. These patients, too, experienced dramatic relief from a variety of unresolved mental and physical complaints.[2]

Dr. Truss hypothesizes that the immune system keeps the yeast in check without difficulty in a healthy person. But certain factors affecting the body's chemistry can drastically upset the balance. *Pregnancy* is one. *Birth control pills* are another. Treatment with *antibiotics* kills the good intestinal bacteria, allowing the yeast to flourish unchecked. *Immunosuppressant drugs,* such as cortisone, weaken the immune system so that the body is no longer able to control the yeast. As the yeast colonies multiply, the weakened immune system is challenged further. The body may regain control naturally—or the yeast may continue to spread.

At this point the person may experience an obvious yeast infection. Vaginal yeast infections cause a thick, lumpy, white discharge with a yeastlike odor and severe itching. Thrush is an oral Candida infection causing mouth soreness and a milklike scum to appear on the tongue, cheeks, and roof of the mouth. If an attempt is made to scrape the scum away, the area may bleed slightly. Candida may also cause skin infections, particularly around and under the nails. However, not everyone suffering from a chronic Candida infection shows these overt symptoms. You may be unaware that you have a yeast infestation.

In other words, a Candida infection can go "underground." Although it doesn't show itself in typical yeast infection symptoms, it may generate other problems. As the yeast colonies multiply, they constantly release a variety of yeast toxins into the bloodstream, paralyzing the immune system. A vicious cycle begins: The yeast multiplies and overwhelms the immune system; the weakened immune system can't control the yeast colonies so they spread.

Let's go back to Dr. Truss's patients.[3] What were some of the dramatic results he reported for his anti-yeast therapy? One 36-year-old woman suffered from severe sinus headaches. She was also schizophrenic and had deteriorated (despite drug and electroshock therapies) to the point where permanent commitment to a state mental hospital had been recommended by her psychiatrist. This woman had been remarkably healthy until age 25, when she developed vaginal and skin fungus infections, which recurred repeatedly. Later, she experienced hormone problems—excessive menstruation and cramps, lack of sexual interest, and premenstrual tension. Then came severe nervousness and depression, along with acute back pain. Amazing as it may sound, treatment with Candida extract relieved all these symptoms. This woman is no longer schizophrenic. Her headaches, backaches, and menstrual problems have disappeared.

A young woman was diagnosed as having multiple sclerosis by her neurologist. She had a long allergy history. Her menstrual cycle had always been abnormal, with severe premenstrual tension. She had also had chronic intestinal and vaginal yeast infection symptoms. From childhood on, antibiotic after antibiotic had been prescribed. Treatment with nystatin for two years brought complete relief. Her symptoms returned after nystatin was stopped, but they disappeared once the drug was started again.

Dr. Crook and dozens of other physicians have now confirmed Dr. Truss's brilliant clinical observations. Dr. Crook has also described a number of children with complex health problems who improved dramatically on anti-yeast therapy. Included among these patients were a six-year-old boy with hyperactivity and a "severe and pervasive developmental disorder" with associated autistic behavior, and several children with recurrent ear infections.[4]

Dr. Truss has also seen many patients with chronic Candida infection who have developed severe intolerances to inhalants, foods, drugs, and chemicals.[5] In fact, the patient who is sensitive to many different substances is the one most likely to respond to anti-yeast therapy. The person who is only ragweed-sensitive or allergic to a few foods is less likely to respond to anti-yeast therapy. In the severe cases, clearing the yeast infection eliminates the multiple intolerances. Recovery may begin within a few weeks of treatment and be complete in several months, or it may take from one to three years, with gradual improvement, in severely affected patients. *Patience* and *persistence* are required!

## ■ CLUES THAT SUGGEST YEAST-RELATED HEALTH PROBLEMS

Other than provocative testing, there is no test as yet to diagnose a Candida infection if it has gone "underground." Still, several positive answers to the following questions suggest you *may* have a Candida problem:

1. Do you have a history of yeast infections—oral, vaginal, or intestinal?
2. Did your symptoms start or get worse after taking birth control pills, antibiotics, or drugs such as cortisone, or after repeated pregnancies?
3. Have you ever taken tetracycline for acne? Have you taken repeated rounds of antibiotics for recurrent bladder, ear, or other infections?

4. Do you suffer from:
   —Various menstrual difficulties (such as spotting, excessive bleeding, cramping, and endometriosis) with symptoms increasing right before or at the beginning of your menstrual period?
   —Diminished sexual interest?
   —Chronic constipation, diarrhea, rectal itching, spastic colon, or mucous colitis?
   —Urgent or frequent urination or prostatitis?
   —Chronic nasal congestion or other respiratory symptoms?
   —Headaches?
   —Muscle aches?
   —Multiple allergies?
   —An auto-immune disorder such as multiple sclerosis, lupus, rheumatoid arthritis, or Crohn's disease?
5. Are you sensitive to molds or baker's and brewer's yeast? (Molds such as Alternaria, Hormodendrum, and Cephalosporum are closely related to Candida.)
6. Does eating refined carbohydrates make your symptoms worse and give you gas and bloating? (Carbohydrates feed the yeast.) Do you feel better on a low-carbohydrate diet?

One helpful way to determine if Candida may be a factor in your problems is to follow a yeast and mold elimination diet (see below), and see if you get better.

## ■ STEPS TO AVOID YEAST

Dr. Truss recommends the following program in treating a chronic Candida infection:[6]

1. Reduce exposure to all yeast foods and their relatives in your diet. Avoid the following foods as much as possible:

—Baked goods raised with baker's yeast.
—Products enriched with vitamins (brewer's yeast).
—Most B-vitamin preparations (a few all-rice bran B-vitamins are available).
—Vinegars and products containing vinegar. (Fresh lemon juice can be used to make salad dressings and mayonnaise.)
—Fermented beverages such as alcoholic beverages, root beer, and ginger ale.
—Mushrooms.
—Foods high in mold content such as aged cheeses, buttermilk, and sour cream. (Plain yogurt, cottage cheese, cream cheese, and processed cheeses are allowed.)
—Malted products such as cereals, candy, and malted milk drinks.
—Citrus juices, unless home squeezed.
—Dried fruits.
—Monosodium glutamate (MSG) and citric acid, which are often yeast derivatives.

2. Begin a low-carbohydrate diet. Yeast colonies cannot live and reproduce well on proteins and fats alone; by depriving them of high levels of carbohydrates you help kill them off. Most Americans consome some 225 grams of carbohydrates each day. Dr. Truss's recommended level for this diet is about 60 to 80 grams per day. If improvement occurs, carbohydrates can be increased.
    a. Buy yourself a pocket carbohydrate counter so you can keep tabs on how much carbohydrate you consume each day. What you'll find is that plain meats have no carbohydrates at all. Neither do vegetable oils. Many vegetables are quite low; fruits and grains are higher. Sugary baked goods and starchy dishes such as macaroni and spaghetti are very high. Consult Ap-

pendix D for the carbohydrate content of some common foods.

b. In setting up your low-carbohydrate diet, take care to ensure adequate nutrition. Since the emphasis will be on vegetables, meats, fish, nuts, a few fresh fruits, and small portions of grains, this shouldn't be difficult—unless you have multiple food allergies. In that case, professional nutritional guidance can be very helpful.

c. Try to master any strong food cravings, especially for carbohydrates. These cravings tend to come and go. Do the best you can in mustering your willpower, but don't feel guilty if you blow your diet. Generally, the Candida-sensitive person feels much better on a low-carbohydrate diet, providing the incentive to continue.

3. Stay away from antibiotics, unless absolutely necessary. Daily antibiotics for acne should be avoided by the Candida-sensitive person. Recently, when my son Jack needed penicillin for a strep throat, it aggravated his yeast problems so much that his accompanying allergy symptoms were worse for months.
4. Avoid contraceptive hormones—that means, the pill. Not every woman on the pill ends up with a Candida problem, but those who do have this problem will be much worse on the pill.
5. Minimize your exposure to high-mold environments (see Chapter 6 for specific steps to take).

## ■ PRESCRIPTION DRUGS USED TO KILL OFF YEAST INFECTIONS

Two anti-yeast prescription drugs are available to reduce the Candida colonies in the body. Nystatin (Mycostatin, Nilstat) is the drug most often used since it is effective and has fewer and less serious side effects (nausea is the most common one). In fact, nystatin is one of the least toxic drugs on the market. It kills only the yeast cells, not the good intestinal bacteria, and only minute amounts of it are absorbed into the bloodstream.[7] Ketaconazole (Nizoral) is the other drug that is sometimes used, but it must be taken with caution. One of its potentially serious side effects is liver inflammation, making monthly liver function tests essential as a precautionary measure.

Nystatin is available in tablets, but the colored coatings often bother the sensitive person. Fortunately, it is now available to your pharmacist or doctor from the drug company in powder form. This powder can be mixed in water or placed in clear gelatin capsules, obtainable from your pharmacist.

Dr. Truss recommends a starting dose of one nystatin tablet (⅛ teaspoon powder) four times a day after meals.[8] If symptoms persist, in three to six weeks the dose is increased to two tablets four times a day. Then, if necessary, this dose may be further increased to three and finally four tablets four times daily. The aim is to relieve symptoms with as low a dose as possible. Some very sensitive patients can't tolerate the starting dosage. An attempt is made to find a dose they can tolerate, even it if seems extremely small. Then, they may be able to gradually increase the amount.

Some doctors use a combination of oral tablets or powder, oral mouthwashes, creams or lotions for yeast skin infections, and vaginal suppositories to destroy as many yeast colonies as possible. They may recommend pills, powders, or liquids containing Lactobacillus acidophilus, the friendly bacteria normally found in yogurt and buttermilk. In your intestines, these friendly bacteria may help crowd out the Candida.

## REBUILDING THE IMMUNE RESPONSE

If your immune response has been weakened, there may be several ways to strengthen it. First of all, make sure that you are eating an adequate diet, with the nutrients necessary for a healthy immune response (see Chapters 10 and 11). Your doctor should be able to rule out (or treat) any medical condition, such as a thyroid imbalance, that impairs the immune response. Also check on any medication you're taking. In particular, immunosuppressant drugs, such as cortisone or prednisone, should be avoided. Although these drugs help suppress allergic reactions, they also help the yeast to thrive. For some people, however, these drugs are life-saving. Then, the dosage must be carefully monitored by a physician, and the risks and benefits carefully weighed.

Treatment with Candida albicans extract may be advisable if your immune system is weak. Two methods are now being used. The first, the one used by Dr. Truss, involves extremely weak injections of Candida extract to help stimulate the body's immune system to fight off the yeast itself. Doses may be gradually increased but never become very strong. The other method uses provocative testing and neutralization with Candida albicans extract. The neutralizing doses tend to be stronger than those in the first method. Immunological studies are currently under way to determine which method is most effective. Researchers are also trying to learn how Candida paralyzes the immune system, how the condition can be accurately diagnosed, and what the best form of therapy really is.[9]

## FINDING HELP FOR YEAST-RELATED ILLNESS

Yeast can normally be found on the membranes lining your body cavities. Yet until Dr. Truss began to publish his pioneer observations in 1978, few physicians realized this common critter could be related to many baffling health problems. Moreover, because the Truss papers cannot be found in every medical library, your physician may not know of this relationship. Yet Candida albicans often plays an important role in aggravating food and chemical sensitivities.

Because no presently available test enables your doctor to identify these yeast-related health problems, diagnosis depends on your history and response to an anti-yeast treatment program. So if you have answered yes to two or more of the six questions listed in the section "Clues That Suggest Yeast-related Health Problems," present your doctor with copies of Dr. Truss's book, *The Missing Diagnosis*, and Dr. Crook's book, *The Yeast Connection*.

# 10

# Improving Your Diet

Many Americans subsist on junk food—high in calories, sugar, fat, and salt, but low in fiber and essential vitamins and minerals. Breakfast is often a cup of coffee, with a midmorning snack of a donut and more coffee. Lunch may be a hamburger, fries, and a milkshake—or maybe a gelatin salad if the person is dieting. For dinner, there's just meat and potatoes. No wonder people's bodies and minds aren't functioning well, that they feel pooped and irritable, or even worse. We are what we eat and drink! With or without allergies, a poor diet may be the cause of physical and psychological problems.

A 1977 study by the United States government concluded that the health of Americans could be vastly improved by a better diet. The statistics cited are staggering. Here are some of the diet-related disorders this study found, along with the number of victims: 25 million people in the U.S. have a mental health disability; 16 million are afflicted with arthritis; 23 million have advanced gum disease and 50% of those over 55 have no teeth; 3.9 million are overtly diabetic and 70% of those over 55 have impaired glucose tolerance; 4

million have severe osteoporosis (a bone disease); 30 to 40% of adults are obese; 5 million are alcoholics; and 32 million have allergies![1]

## THE SUGAR PROBLEM

Remember my earlier remarks about the dangers of sugar (in Chapter 2)? Well, the average American consumes about one-half cup of sugar each day, or more than 100 pounds per year.[2] Picture that as twenty 5-pound bags of sugar overflowing a grocery cart. It's an astonishing amount!

You may not think you eat much sugar, but have you considered the sugar content of prepared foods? Some presweetened breakfast cereals contain as much as 50% sugar. Catsup may be 10% sugar. Less obvious sources of sugar are soups, yogurt, luncheon meats, canned or frozen vegetables and fruits, breads, peanut butter, and salad dressings. Even table salt may have some dextrose, which is added to help it flow freely. In fact, 15% to 20% of the average American diet is refined sugar.[3]

There's no denying that sugar tastes great. And our sweet tooths may be inborn. If a sugar solution is injected into the fluid surrounding an unborn child, the fetus will immediately begin to swallow the sweet fluid.[4] Infants may come into contact with sugar as early as the first day of life, if they're fed sugar water while the mother is waiting for her milk to come in. Sweetened infant formulas and baby foods help perpetuate a sweet tooth.

There are a lot of reasons to cut down on your sugar intake. Recall that sugar is mostly empty calories. Eating sugary foods may keep you from getting essential vitamins and minerals; it may even increase your body's need for certain vitamins and minerals just to process the sugar. Sugar also interferes with maintaining a stable blood sugar level. And allergy victims may encounter special problems with sugar—they may even have allergic reactions to the sugar they buy (see Chapter 2). Moreover, the refined carbohydrates in high-sugar foods tend to intensify symptoms in people with Candida infections (see Chapter 9).

And have you thought about the possibility of dental decay? Some dentists estimate that as many as 95% of American children have active dental decay,[5] and they are concerned that dental decay may be a systemic disease, an overt sign of a body whose chemistry is out of wack. Sugar plays an important role in causing tooth decay. Experiments have shown that even when rats are fed sugar solutions via stomach tubes or by injection—with no contact with the teeth—they develop dental decay at the same rate as rats who eat the same amount of sugar by mouth![6] Another problem is that cavities are usually filled with a silver preparation containing mercury. Some concerned dentists report that a hypersensitivity to mercury may set up a whole host of allergies and other symptoms (see Chapter 12).

Whether you decide to eliminate sugar from your diet entirely may depend on the severity of your symptoms. Although total avoidance is the ideal and may be necessary for some individuals, it's not easy to accomplish. Some people find that once they've totally given up sugar, any time they eat it they feel miserable. Others find that by cutting it out most of the time, they can cheat occasionally without symptoms. Still others have discovered that just a reduced sugar consumption improves their symptoms. But whatever you decide to do, remember that sugar is addictive. If you are a "sugarholic" and stop eating sugar cold turkey, you will probably experience uncomfortable withdrawal symptoms—headaches, depression, and fatigue. Cut back gradually.

What can you use instead of sugar to satisfy your sweet cravings? First of all, you won't crave sugar as much if you don't eat it. A little bit of sugar often just makes you want more. But if your sweet tooth persists, small amounts of honey and pure maple syrup can be used to satisfy it. Be sure to buy your honey from a reliable local source so that you know it hasn't been diluted with corn syrup. Of course, if you start substituting lots of honey and maple syrup for all the sugar, you're not going to be any further ahead. Their nutrients are minimal; both are high in calories; and they, too, can affect your blood sugar levels and promote tooth decay. Moreover, allergy to honey and maple syrup does occur. Certainly, it's not a magical solution. But honey and pure maple syrup, used sparingly, can help make the transition easier from high-sugar foods to natural, unsweetened foods. Adding chopped naturally sweet fruits, such as apples, pineapples, dates, bananas, raisins, and oranges, may help you reduce or eliminate sugar in recipes (see Chapter 15 for recipe suggestions). Eaten whole, these fruits make great snacks and desserts. While satisfying your cravings for sweets, they are also nutritious.

Should you try an artificial sweetener? Saccharin may be a temporary solution to ease your sweet cravings, but by and large it should be avoided. All saccharin products carry a warning that it may be detrimental to your health. Saccharin also reinforces the idea that things have to taste sweet to taste good, and it has no nutritional benefits. Some people are allergic to saccharin; they may experience a wide variety of symptoms but often the culprit—the artificial sweetener—goes unsuspected.

The new low-calorie sweetener aspartame (Equal) seems to be an improvement over saccharin. It's made from protein components similar to those found naturally in many foods, and underwent vigorous safety testing before its approval by the Food and Drug Administration. Although low in calories, it tastes sweet, with no bitter aftertaste. It is, however, mixed with milk sugar (lactose), which may bother some milk-sensitive persons. And whether highly allergic people will react to the materials from which it is derived remains to be seen. (See Chapter 15 for recipe suggestions using aspartame.)

## SOME OTHER "NO-NOS"

You've probably already heard about the dangers of too much caffeine. This addictive substance is found not only in coffee, but also in cocoa, chocolate, cola beverages, many kinds of tea, and some headache remedies. Caffeine is a stimulant so it temporarily "perks you up" by increasing mental alertness and lessening fatigue. But be aware that too much caffeine may lead to a variety of symptoms, including anxiety, irregular heartbeat, headache, and irritability. The threshold for caffeine tolerance varies from person to person. Some people are allergic to caffeine itself; others are sensitive to foods containing caffeine.

As with sugar, suddenly cutting caffeine out of your diet may cause severe withdrawal symptoms. A gradual reduction is usually more successful. If you're a coffee addict, start by mixing regular coffee with decaffeinated coffee, gradually reducing the amount of caffeine. Or try some caffeine-free herb teas. Concentrated unsweetened fruit juices mixed with bubbly spring water or club soda can replace soft drinks. Carob is a delicious chocolate-substitute and can be used in baking and beverages (see Chapter 19).

Here's another un-American idea. If you think you're promoting your health by drinking milk, you may be dead-wrong. Cow's milk is a super-food—but for calves, not humans. Adults do not need milk if their diet is otherwise adequate. After all, humans prospered for thousands of years before they began to drink cow's milk. Many people—some 10 to 30% of the world population—lack the necessary enzyme to digest milk properly, causing intestinal symptoms.[7] And if you drink lots of milk, which is very filling, you may not have room left for other nutritious foods. Although milk is rich in calcium and vitamins A, D, and $B_{12}$, it lacks iron, vitamin C, most B vitamins, and manganese. Moreover, some evidence suggests that calcium in cow's milk is hard to absorb.[8] So milk is not the perfect food—in fact, no one food is. It may even be that you are sensitive to cow's milk, as this is an extremely common food allergen. If so, chances are that you'll feel better and be healthier on a milk-reduced or milk-free diet.

Yet another thing to limit is your intake of food additives. Not all additives are bad, however (see Appendix C). What you need to avoid are products with artificial colorings and flavorings, monosodium glutamate (MSG), and preservatives (BHA, BHT, and nitrites). These particular additives often present problems for sensitive individuals. Moreover, food containing these additives are usually nutritionally deficient and highly processed. Substitute unprocessed products.

And what about alcohol? Although, for many people, an alcoholic drink or two occasionally is probably harmless (and maybe even beneficial), larger amounts affect the blood sugar level, add empty calories to the diet, and can be a potent allergen. Even in small amounts, alcoholic beverages are poorly tolerated by Candida-sensitive people. If you feel you must have a drink to be social, try a glass of bubbly spring water with a twist of lime—it's refreshing and harmless!

## ■ STEPS TOWARD A HEALTHY DIET

So far we've looked at all the things you shouldn't do. What positive steps can you take to guarantee an adequate diet? Here are some basic guidelines.

1. Use wholewheat or wholewheat pastry flour, preferably stone-ground. Bleaching and maturing agents affect some sensitive persons, and many important nutrients are lost completely when wheat is refined. If you don't like the texture of wholewheat for all your baking needs, use unbleached white flour and add either wholewheat flour or wheat germ to increase the nutritional value. Also select stone-ground cornmeal, rye, and brown rice flours. Use whole brown rice, not white rice.
2. Choose fresh fruits and vegetables when possible. Frozen products are less desirable but better than canned. Raw fruits and vegetables are preferred; if you do cook them, keep the cooking time short to preserve the nutritional value.
3. Select lean meats, poultry, and fish. Try nuts, legumes, and seeds to replace some of the animal protein in your diet. Soybeans are nutritious and cheap.
4. Vary your diet as much as possible—it's the best way to ensure adequate nutrition. As a quick recap, here are some suggestions on what to choose (or not choose):
   a. *Best foods:*
      —Whole-grain cereals, brown rice.
      —Bread made from stone-ground grains.
      —A variety of raw fresh vegetables, especially dark green, leafy vegetables.
      —Raw fresh fruit.
      —Cold-pressed, pure vegetable oils.

—Yogurt (without sugar), cottage cheese (no additives), butter; but only if you're not milk-sensitive.
—Nuts and seeds (raw, unprocessed).
—Beans, sprouts.
—Eggs.
—Seafood, chicken, turkey, rabbit.

b. *Other good foods:*
—Pure fruit and vegetable juices.
—Cooked vegetables and fruits.
—Lean beef and pork.
—Small amounts of dried fruits (no preservatives).
—Small amounts of pure honey and pure maple syrup.

c. *Foods to avoid:*
—Refined sugar.
—Bleached white flour.
—White rice.
—Artificial colorings, flavorings, MSG, preservatives.
—Presweetened cereals.
—Canned vegetables and fruits, especially in syrups.
—Ham, luncheon meats, hot dogs.
—Coffee, most teas, chocolate.
—Soft drinks.
—Candy.
—Processed snack food.
—Artificial sweeteners (saccharin).

These are difficult steps to take in the average American family. Several months may be required to make the transition from junk foods to a nutritious diet. Very few people can stick to this diet 100% of the time. But do the best you can! The dividends will last a lifetime.

# 11

# Overcoming Nutritional Deficiencies

The use of vitamins and minerals to alleviate various physical and mental symptoms is extremely controversial. Most of the medical "establishment" declares that anyone who eats a good, balanced diet needs no additional vitamins or minerals. If you ask your doctor if you should take a daily multivitamin preparation, he or she may answer that although the only thing it will hurt is your pocketbook, it won't make you healthier. And if you ask if larger doses might be helpful for depression or allergies, your doctor may dismiss you as "one of those health food nuts" and give you a lecture on the harmful effects of too many vitamins.

On the other side of this heated debate is a group of doctors who claim they have found a whole new approach to psychiatric and medical problems through using large doses of nutrients to compensate for biochemical imbalances. In the middle, as usual, is the patient—not knowing what to believe but anxious to get well.

What is a vitamin, and why is there all this controversy? A vitamin is an organic substance found in plants and animals in varying quantities. Each different vitamin is absolutely necessary for proper growth and maintenance of health. Except for a few vitamins, your body cannot make these chemicals itself. You must obtain them from your diet or in vitamin supplements.

Six basic nutrients are essential for life: carbohydrates, fats, proteins, vitamins, minerals, and water. If you think of your body as a car engine, carbohydrates, fats, and proteins are the gasoline giving you energy. But vitamins are the spark plugs, oil, and grease; without their presence, your body can't function. They are the catalysts for all the biochemical reactions in your body.

There are two kinds of vitamins: fat-soluble and water-soluble. Fat-soluble A, D, E, and K vitamins dissolve only in fat and are therefore stored by the body. Taken in excess, they can be harmful. Water-soluble B-complex and C vitamins dissolve in water so that excess amounts not needed by the body are excreted in the urine. But these vitamins must be obtained daily.

Vitamins were isolated and identified during the first half of this century. Considerable interest and enthusiasm were aroused by their ability to cure deficiency diseases such as scurvy and beriberi. But when antibiotics began to crowd the scene in the 1940s, catching all the attention, excitement over vitamins diminished. To safeguard our health, the Food and Nutrition Board of the National Academy of Sciences was established in 1941. They came up with a list of minimum daily nutrient requirements, which has been revised over the years and is now referred to as the Recommended Dietary Allowance (RDA).

The RDA opens up one aspect of the controversy. Nutritionally oriented doctors agree with the medical establishment that following the RDA will generally prevent vitamin-deficiency diseases. Where they disagree is on whether this is a good guideline for everybody. These nutritionally oriented doctors believe there is an optimal dosage of each nutrient for each person that allows that person to function physically and mentally at his or her best. In their opinion, an average value (such as the RDA) doesn't consider that each person is biochemically unique. They contend that a variety of factors determine how much of a given nutrient a person needs, including height and weight, age, activity level, stress, smoking, alcohol intake, use of birth control pills, pregnancy, breast-feeding, infection, and such environmental conditions as air pollution.

What especially concerns these doctors is that not only do many Americans not eat a good diet (see Chapter 10) but they also don't really know what a good diet is. And traditional medical education may be as much to blame as anything. As the old story goes, the average doctor probably knows a little more about nutrition than the average secretary, unless the secretary is on a diet—in which case, the secretary probably knows more! Preliminary results of a nationwide survey of food consumption conducted by the U.S. Department of Agriculture indicate that many Americans are deficient in six of the 12 essential nutrients studied: calcium, iron, magnesium, vitamin A, vitamin $B_6$, and vitamin C. Women and teenage girls were particularly deficient, often lacking more than 30% of the RDA.[1]

Nutritionally oriented doctors are also concerned that modern processing of whole foods robs the consumer of essential nutrients, even though manufacturers attempt to undo the damage by enriching their products with a few essential vitamins and minerals.

Perhaps the most emotional issue is the use of megavitamins—large doses of certain vitamins to prevent and treat physical and mental problems. Whether or not large doses of vitamin C, for instance, will help prevent colds or ease their severity is hotly debated. Although the RDA of vitamin C for adults is 60 milligrams, large doses used to prevent colds and infections may range from 250 milligrams to 10,000 milligrams per day.

Part of the controversy centers on the question of safety. How safe are megavitamins? The medical establishment declares they may be hazardous to your health. They're concerned about self-medicating by people who don't really know what they're doing, especially as large doses of fat-soluble vitamins can cause severe symptoms. And they're worried that some patients will figure if they take their vitamins, it doesn't matter what they eat or do. Perhaps these patients will ignore early warning signs of serious disease, opting for vitamins instead of seeking medical attention. But beyond this, the medical establishment tends to see megavitamin therapy as a faddish "trick," even when it's practiced by experienced medical doctors.

Obviously, nutritionally oriented doctors share some of these safety concerns. But they also believe that megavitamin therapy, if properly handled, is much safer than many conventional medications and more effective. In their opinion, the medical establishment has a closed mind; it's condemning—without investigating—a valid treatment.

So where does this leave you, the frustrated patient? What I'd advise is based on my own experience, spending years looking for the best answers to help my family. Balancing your body chemistry is complicated. *Find an experienced orthomolecular or nutritionally oriented doctor or dentist to help you.* Such a doctor can save you lots of time and money in the long run by closely monitoring symptoms, diet, and hair, blood, and urine levels of various nutrients. Definitely do not blindly dose yourself with vitamins and minerals without professional guidance. It's wrong to think: "If one pill makes me feel better, ten pills will help even more." You may make yourself worse. And be wary of taking a single vitamin or mineral over a long period of time. Nutrients interact with each other and taking large doses of one may cause deficiencies of others. As one expert sums it up: "Megadoses have been used in the medical field for some years with great results, but leave the big bullets to the big guns. Leave it for those who have experience and evidence for what they are doing."[2]

If someone recommends that you take so much of such and such vitamin, be sure the information is reliable. I've been appalled at some of the practices I've seen in health food stores. One salesperson offered my children vitamin pills as though they were candy: "Here, kids, you'll love the taste, and it's good for you." Another time a salesperson was pushing chewable vitamin C tablets at the checkout counter. She told the woman ahead of me to try one of the samples. When the woman remarked how tasty it was, the salesperson sold her a large bottle with the advice: "Eat them all day, they can't possibly harm you, and they'll give you so much energy." She neglected to mention to the unsuspecting customer that too much vitamin C can cause gas and diarrhea!

What about the issue of synthetic vitamins versus organic ones? Natural vitamins are supposed to be made by concentrating the vitamins as they occur naturally in plant and animal sources. Synthetic vitamins are derived by taking other chemicals and changing them into chemicals having the same structures as the natural vitamin forms. Some say the results are identical; others say that natural vitamins are much better. In some cases, such as pantothenic acid, the cost of the natural form is prohibitive and a synthetic source is the only practical solution. In general, natural vitamins are much more expensive than synthetic ones. Some doctors think your chances of reacting adversely are greater with synthetic vitamins, but it's not uncommon to be allergic to the source of natural vitamins, such as fish oil or brewer's yeast.

Another problem is the fillers, binders, dyes, and flavorings used. Generally, synethetic vitamins seem to contain more of these, but you may have similar trouble with natural vitamins, too. You'll have to read the labels. If you can't obtain this information from the bottle, contact the manufacturer. Appendix B lists some manufacturers who make an effort to avoid common allergy-causing materials and who will provide you with a list of the contents for each of their products.

By now you're probably wondering how to get more information on specific nutrients. Most of the rest of this chapter focuses on various nutrients that have been found to be helpful for allergies and associated problems. *Keep in mind the pitfalls of self-dosing.* Look for a doctor or dentist who is well-trained in this area and is interested in helping you find the doses that are right for *you.* Appendix B gives addresses for organizations that will help you find a doctor or dentist in your area.

## ■ GETTING A GOOD VITAMIN SUPPLY

### Vitamin A

Vitamin A is important for the development of bones and teeth and essential to maintaining healthy skin cells and mucous membranes. It aids in the growth and repair of body tissues and plays an important role in the immune system in fighting infections. Vitamin A is essential for good eyesight and night vision. In checking for the adequacy of your vitamin A supply, however, remember that vitamin A is a fat-soluble vitamin—if you take too much, it is stored in your body fat and can cause serious problems.

To see if you *might* be deficient in vitamin A, ask yourself the following questions. Several positive answers would suggest this possibility—but remember, it's only a possibility.

1. Are you pregnant or breast-feeding?
2. Have you recently been ill? Do you have frequent infections?
3. Are you under a lot of stress?
4. Do you smoke and/or live in an area of high air pollution?
5. Do you take mineral oil often? (Mineral oil depletes your supply of all fat-soluble vitamins and should be avoided.)
6. Have you experienced trouble seeing at night? Are your eyes very sensitive to sunlight? Do you have any other eye problems?
7. Is your skin rough, dry, or scaly? Do you have acne? Goose bumps?
8. Do you work in an area with excessively bright or dim lights?

The adult RDA (age 15 up) for vitamin A is 5,000 International Units for men and 4,000 IU for women. Pregnancy and nursing increases the body's need. Vitamin A is derived from carotene, a pigment found in abundance in orange-colored fruits and vegetables, and in dark green leafy vegetables. It is stable under ordinary cooking temperatures. Some good dietary sources are:

| | |
|---|---|
| Beef liver (4 ounces) | 60,500 IU[3] |
| Carrot (1 large) | 11,000 |

| | |
|---|---|
| Spinach (1 cup cooked) | 8,100 |
| Sweet potato (1 small) | 8,100 |
| Pumpkin (½ cup, canned) | 8,000 |
| Cantaloupe (½ medium) | 6,500 |
| Broccoli (1 cup, cooked) | 3,750 |
| Peach (1 medium) | 1,516 |
| Tomato (1 medium) | 1,390 |
| Apricot (1 medium) | 1,026 |
| Butter or margarine (1 tablespoon) | 462 |
| Whole milk (1 cup, fortified) | 354 |

Vitamin A supplements are available in cod liver oil (1 tablespoon = 35,000 IU), capsules of fish liver oil, carrot oil, and lemon grass, as well as water-soluble tablets of synthetic vitamin A palmitate or acetate. Do not, as an adult, exceed doses of 25,000 IU without the supervision of a knowledgeable physician. Do not give vitamin A supplements to children or babies unless your doctor prescribes them.

Symptoms of taking too much vitamin A include hair loss, nausea, vomiting, diarrhea, bone pain, headaches, scaly skin, fatigue, liver enlargement, and mental disorders such as depression.

### Vitamin B-Complex

The B-complex vitamins include several different water-soluble compounds, which are grouped together by scientists because they work together in your body. The whole B family should be supplemented, not just one member. B vitamins are vital for the breakdown of carbohydrates, fats, and proteins into energy. They are also essential for a healthy nervous system and for healthy hair, skin, eyes, mouth, and liver. In addition, B vitamins assist in the production of antibodies and red blood cells, as well as the regulation of body fluids.

Use the following questions to see if you *might* be

lacking in B vitamins. Again, however, several positive replies only *suggest* this possibility.

1. Do you take birth control pills? Or are you pregnant or breast-feeding?
2. Are you under stress? Do you get frequent infections?
3. Do you smoke? Use alcohol and caffeine regularly?
4. Is your carbohydrate intake high?
5. Are you often tired, irritable, and depressed? Is your appetite poor? Do you suffer from insomnia?
6. Do you have skin problems such as oiliness, itching, or burning? Scaly sores? Cracks at the corners of your mouth? Stretch marks on your hips and thighs? Dandruff on your scalp or eyebrows?
7. Is your tongue enlarged—shiny, bright red, and full of grooves? Is it cracked and sore?
8. Do you have little or no dream recall?
9. Are you oversensitive to noise and light?
10. Have your menstrual periods been irregular? Do you experience premenstrual tension? Retain water easily?
11. Do you have low blood sugar?

Here are the RDAs (in milligrams) for some of the B-complex vitamins:

| | *Men* | *Women* |
|---|---|---|
| *Thiamine ($B_1$)* | *1.2–1.5 mgs* | *1.0–1.1 mgs* |
| Riboflavin ($B_2$) | 1.4–1.7 | 1.2–1.3 |
| Niacin | 16–19 | 13–14 |
| Pyridoxine ($B_6$) | 2.0–2.2 | 2.0 |
| Folic acid | .4 | .4 |
| Pantothenic acid | Not set | |
| $B_{12}$ | .003 | .003 |

B-complex vitamins are easily destroyed—some by heat and light; some by food processing. Chart 5 shows some natural dietary sources for your B-complex vitamin supply.

The B-complex vitamins available in capsules or tablets are derived from yeast, rice, or synthetic sources. Supplements that provide around 25 milligrams of thiamine, niacin, and $B_6$ plus all the other B vitamins are usually safe and adequate. Because the B-complex vitamins are water-soluble, excess amounts are excreted in the urine.

Nevertheless, excess amounts of *one* of the B vitamins taken over a period of time may cause deficiencies in the other B vitamins. Megadoses of B vitamins should be taken under the care of an experienced physician since side effects are possible. Excessive amounts of folic acid, for instance, can mask a $B_{12}$ deficiency. Too much $B_{12}$ can lower your folic acid level. Niacin in large doses can cause an intense flushing of the skin. Although this flushing reaction passes quickly and is harmless, it may be uncomfortable and scary if you're unprepared. Niacinamide, another form of this vitamin, does not cause this flushing but may cause nausea. Large doses of $B_6$ may cause restlessness at night or excessive dream recall. $B_6$ also acts as a diuretic and may deplete the body of essential trace minerals. Riboflavin turns the urine yellow—a harmless side effect.

### Vitamin C

Vitamin C increases the transport of many nutrients through the cell membrane. It is important for the formation of blood vessels, red blood cells, bones, teeth, and—especially—connective tissues (thus helping to heal wounds and burns). It is also believed to fight bacterial and viral infections and to reduce the

**CHART 5. Food Sources for B-Complex Vitamins (in milligrams)**

| *Food* | *Thiamine* | *Riboflavin* | *Niacin* | *Pyridoxine* | *Folic Acid* | *Pantothenic Acid* | $B_{12}$ |
|---|---|---|---|---|---|---|---|
| Beef liver (4 ounces) | .3 | 4.7 | 18.7 | .9 | .35 | 8.7 | — |
| Brewer's yeast (1 tablespoon) | 1.6 | .42 | 3.8 | .2 | .2 | 1.1 | — |
| Wheat germ (1 tablespoon) | .16 | .04 | .25 | .06 | .01 | .10 | — |
| Wholewheat flour (1 cup) | .66 | .14 | 5.16 | 1.12 | .05 | 1.3 | — |
| Pork roast (4 ounces) | .58 | .26 | 4.5 | — | — | — | — |
| Milk (1 cup) | .07 | .42 | .24 | .09 | .002 | .75 | .98 |
| Peanuts (½ cup) | .38 | .16 | 20.0 | .35 | .07 | 2.88 | — |
| Spinach (1 cup, steamed) | .07 | .14 | .5 | .13 | .075 | .07 | — |
| Yogurt (1 cup, plain) | .1 | .45 | .25 | .012 | — | .78 | .28 |
| Egg (1 medium) | .06 | .15 | .05 | .06 | .003 | .80 | 1.00 |

effects on the body of allergy-causing substances.

Again, if you find yourself giving several "yes" answers to the following questions, you *may* be lacking in vitamin C.

1. Do you smoke and/or live in an area of high air pollution?
2. Are you under stress? Do you have frequent infections?
3. Do you take birth control pills, aspirin, antibiotics, or cortisone?
4. Have you been exposed to toxic metals such as lead, mercury, and cadmium?
5. Do you suffer from fatigue, confusion, and depression?
6. Are your gums puffy and spongy, and do they bleed easily?
7. Do you bruise easily? Are your wounds slow to heal?
8. Have you been diagnosed as having iron-deficiency anemia?

The RDA for vitamin C is 60 milligrams for adults, both men and women. Pregnant and nursing women require an extra 20 to 40 milligrams. Citrus fruits are especially high in vitamin C, but other fruits and vegetables also have high quantities. Because vitamin C is easily destroyed by heat, sunlight, air, drying, and long storage, you should, if possible, buy fresh produce and eat the foods raw. Bioflavonoids, water-soluble compounds found in fruits and vegetables containing vitamin C, are essential for the proper use of vitamin C. They are much more concentrated in the whole edible part of the fruit than in the juice. Some good natural sources of vitamin C are:

| | |
|---|---|
| Orange (1 medium) | 90 mgs |
| Broccoli (½ cup) | 68 |
| Orange juice (½ cup, fresh) | 60 |
| Strawberries (¾ cup) | 66 |
| Cantaloupe (½ medium) | 66 |
| Brussels sprouts (½ cup, cooked) | 57 |

| | |
|---|---|
| Grapefruit (½ medium) | 53 |
| Tangerine (1 medium) | 35 |
| Cauliflower (½ cup, steamed) | 33 |
| Beef liver (4 ounces) | 31 |
| Cabbage (½, shredded raw) | 22 |

Most vitamin C supplements are made from corn. They are available in liquids (beware of sugar, colorings, and flavorings), chewable tablets (same problems), timed-release capsules, tablets, and powder. Vitamin C also comes in different forms—ascorbic acid, calcium ascorbate, and sodium ascorbate. Large doses of ascorbic acid may be irritating. Sodium ascorbate may be the best-absorbed but should not be used by those on a sodium-restricted diet.

Taking 2,000 to 3,000 milligrams of vitamin C daily appears to be safe. Nausea, gas, and diarrhea are the signs that you are taking too much and should reduce your dosage slightly. Sudden stoppage of large doses of vitamin C may increase your susceptibility to infection, so reduce large doses gradually. Several grams of vitamin C daily may affect the measurement of glucose in the blood, falsely elevating the level slightly. Theoretically, megadoses of vitamin C may cause kidney stones, but clinical studies have not demonstrated this side effect.

### Vitamin D

Vitamin D is necessary for proper utilization of dietary calcium and phosphorus for strong bones and teeth. It is often called the "sunshine vitamin" because your body manufactures vitamin D when ultraviolet sunlight activates certain chemicals in your skin. Because vitamin D is fat-soluble, it is stored by your body for those days when you can't be outdoors. In those who don't get enough sunshine and don't drink vitamin D-fortified milk, a deficiency may develop. But taking excessive vitamin D supplements over a long period of time can produce serious toxic reactions, as too much accumulates in the body.

Once again, several positive replies to the following questions *may* indicate a lack of vitamin D.

1. Do you take mineral oil?
2. Are you living in an area of high smog? Do you work at night or avoid sunlight? Are you dark-skinned?
3. Do you suffer from bone (osteomalacia, rickets) and tooth problems?

The RDA for vitamin D is 400 International Units. In addition to sunlight, the following are natural sources of vitamin D:

| | |
|---|---|
| Fortified milk (1 cup) | 100 IU |
| Sardines (4 ounces, canned in oil) | 338 |
| Tuna (4 ounces, canned in oil, drained) | 295 |
| Beef liver (4 ounces) | 39 |
| Egg yolk (1) | 27 |
| Butter (1 tablespoon) | 13 |

Vitamin D supplements are available in natural form from fish liver oil or in synthetic form from irradiated ergosterol and calciferol. Don't take doses larger than the RDA of 400 IU unless you are under close medical supervision. Symptoms of taking too much vitamin D are weight loss, nausea, diarrhea, kidney damage, and high blood levels of calcium and phosphorus, leading to calcification of soft tissues.

**Vitamin E**

Vitamin E prevents oxidation of other important vitamins, nutrients, and hormones. There is some controversy over its other functions, but it may play a role in forming normal tissues, promoting the healing of wounds, preventing blood clots, lowering blood pressure, and activating the immune system, as well as protecting against the effects of air pollution. Although vitamin E is fat-soluble, unlike vitamins A and D, the body stores vitamin E for relatively shorter periods of time so large doses are less likely to cause toxic side effects.

In considering if you *might* need more vitamin E, count your affirmative responses to the following questions.

1. Is your diet high in polyunsaturated oils?
2. Do you take iron supplements? (Iron destroys vitamin E so they should not be taken together.)
3. Do you take mineral oils?
4. Are you pregnant, breast-feeding, or going through menopause?
5. Do you live in an area of high air pollution?

The RDA for vitamin E is 10 milligrams for men and 8 milligrams for women. Vitamin E is found in cold-pressed vegetable oils, but is destroyed if the oils are refined, hydrogenated, or heated to a high temperature. Natural dietary sources include:

| | |
|---|---|
| Wheat germ oil (1 tablespoon) | 28.0 mgs |
| Cold-pressed safflower oil (1 tablespoon) | 13.0 |
| Cold-pressed peanut oil (1 tablespoon) | 8.5 |
| Cold-pressed corn oil (1 tablespoon) | 5.0 |
| Wheat germ (1 tablespoon) | 1.8 |

Vitamin E (tocopherol) occurs in several molecular forms. D-alpha tocopherol is the most potent, but supplements of mixed natural tocopherols are probably best. Supplements are derived from soy and wheat germ oils. Too much vitamin E may increase the effect of anticoagulant drugs, leading to excessive bleeding. In high blood pressure patients, large doses of vitamin

E may elevate the pressure. Other milder side effects may be headache, fatigue, and nausea.

## ■ CHECKING YOUR INTAKE OF MINERALS

Minerals are inorganic chemicals. Some, like calcium and magnesium, are needed by your body in fairly large amounts; others are needed in small but critical amounts. Still other minerals, like lead and mercury, can be very toxic inside your body (see Chapter 12).

As with vitamins, deficiencies of certain minerals can cause mild to severe symptoms. Too much of a good mineral can be devastating too. How does your doctor know if you're getting enough or too much of a particular mineral? One way is to order a blood and urine analysis for each mineral. A controversial new technique is hair mineral analysis, which is relatively inexpensive. Some doctors and dentists believe this test can detect abnormal mineral levels before such changes appear in the blood or urine. All that is required is a tablespoon or two of hair from the nape of the neck, clipped close to the scalp. Some labs will run this test without a physician's order; others will not (see Appendix B for labs that do hair analyses). You should, however, find a doctor or dentist who is experienced in interpreting these tests as the results and courses of treatment can be confusing to the layperson. For instance, a mineral deficiency in your body may show up as an excess of the same mineral in your hair! Such results need to be added to those from blood chemistries to make the correct diagnosis. A deficiency of several minerals, for instance, may also indicate a deficiency of hydrochloric acid, insufficient pancreatic enzymes, or an improper balance of intestinal bacteria.

**Calcium**

Calcium, the most abundant mineral in your body, is primarily located in your bones and teeth. In addition to its role in growth, it is essential for normal nervous system functioning, a normal heart rhythm, and blood clotting. It also aids in utilizing iron and helps in the transport of nutrients in and out of cells. Vitamin D is required before the body can use calcium. A proper balance must also be maintained with phosphorus and magnesium.

"Yes" replies to the following questions *plus* results from hair and blood tests may indicate a calcium deficiency.

1. Do you have:
   —Muscle cramps or menstrual cramps?
   —Brittle fingernails?
   —Heart palpitations?
   —Insomnia and nervousness?
2. Are your bones porous and brittle?
3. Are you pregnant or breast-feeding?

The RDA for calcium in men and women is 800 to 1,200 milligrams. Pregnant or breast-feeding women need an extra 400 milligrams daily. Natural dietary sources of calcium include:

| | |
|---|---|
| Almonds (1 cup) | 328 mgs |
| Yogurt (1 cup) | 300 |
| Milk (1 cup) | 287 |
| Cottage cheese (1 cup) | 212 |
| Peanuts (1 cup) | 173 |
| Soybeans (1 cup, cooked) | 146 |
| Spinach (1 cup, cooked) | 93 |

Many different kinds of calcium supplements are available. Bonemeal (dried pulverized cattle bones), oyster shells, and dolomite (ground-up limestone) are often poorly absorbed and may be sources of inactive calcium that the body cannot use.[4] Calcium lactate (from milk), gluconate, chelate, and proteinate are better absorbed. Calcium supplementation must be carefully balanced with magnesium, zinc, and phosphorus intake. Too much calcium may lead to excessive calcification of bones and soft tissues.

### Magnesium

Although, like calcium, magnesium is concentrated in the bones and teeth, it is also present in all body tissues, where it is essential for metabolic processes. Much remains to be learned about magnesium's role, but it is thought to help maintain the body's acid-alkaline balance, assist in blood sugar metabolism, and facilitate normal nerve and muscle functioning. A proper calcium–magnesium balance must be maintained.

If you have several positive replies to the following questions, as well as low levels of magnesium on hair and blood tests, you *may* be deficient in magnesium.

1. Do you suffer from:
   —Confusion, disorientation, nervousness, or hyperactivity?
   —Muscle twitches or tremors?
   —Gum disease?
2. Are you pregnant or breast-feeding?

The RDA for magnesium is 350 to 400 milligrams for men, 300 milligrams for women, 450 milligrams for pregnant or lactating women. Its natural dietary sources include:

| | |
|---|---|
| Peanuts (1 cup) | 420 mgs |
| Almonds (1 cup) | 378 |
| Avocado (1 large) | 97 |

| | |
|---|---|
| Tuna (4 ounces in oil, drained) | 75 |
| Banana (1 medium) | 49 |
| Green beans (1 cup, cooked) | 40 |
| Milk (1 cup, whole milk) | 37 |
| Wheat germ (1 tablespoon) | 19 |
| Wholewheat bread (1 slice) | 18 |
| Apple (1 medium) | 10 |

Magnesium is available in supplements as magnesium oxide, sulfate, or palmitate. Excessive magnesium may be toxic if the calcium intake is deficient and the phosphorus intake is high.

### Zinc

Zinc, an essential trace mineral, is often deficient in our diets because of overprocessing. Zinc is necessary for protein synthesis and carbohydrate digestion. It combines with many enzymes as an essential part of their structure. In addition, zinc plays a role in healing wounds, the normal functioning of the prostate gland, and sex organ growth and development.

Again, combined with low levels of zinc in hair and blood analyses, several "yes" answers to the following questions *may* indicate a zinc deficiency.

1. Do you have:
   —White spots or white banding on your fingernails or toenails?
   —Poor appetite and loss of taste?
   —Gum disease?
   —Prostate problems?
   —Stretch marks on your hips, thighs, abdomen, breast, or shoulders?
   —Brittle hair, lacking pigment?
   —Slow hair and nail growth?
2. Are your wounds slow to heal?

The RDA for zinc for male and female adults is 15 milligrams. Pregnant woman require an extra 5 milligrams; lactating women, an extra 10 milligrams. Good dietary sources are:

| | |
|---|---|
| Oysters (3 ounces) | 143.0 mgs[5] |
| Herrings (3 ounces) | 100.0 |
| Wheat germ (3 ounces) | 13.3 |
| Beef (3 ounces) | 6.4 |
| Beef liver (3 ounces) | 5.5 |
| Peas (3 ounces) | 4.0 |
| Carrots (3 ounces) | 2.0 |
| Egg (1 medium) | 1.5 |
| Wholewheat bread (3 ounces) | 1.04 |

Zinc supplements are available as zinc sulfate, zinc gluconate, and chelated zinc. Taking too much zinc interferes with normal levels of copper, iron, and manganese.

**Iron**

We're all familiar with the TV ads showing tired women suffering from "iron-poor blood" or iron-deficiency anemia. Iron is essential for making red blood cells and certain enzymes. It aids growth, helps resist disease, and helps prevent fatigue.

Positive answers to the following questions *may* suggest you are deficient in iron—but they are only preliminary clues. Before reaching for a bottle of iron pills, consult your doctor for a blood test to see if you are really anemic. The symptoms are similar to many other illnesses and deficiencies. If you are anemic, your doctor will want to determine why.

1. Are you pale? Do you have a poor memory, depression, dizziness, weakness, and fatigue?
2. Are your nails brittle, flattened, and lusterless? Have you had any hair loss?

3. Is your tongue inflamed?
4. Do you suffer from constipation?
5. Do you have excessive menstrual bleeding?

The RDA for iron is 10 to 18 milligrams for men and women. Pregnant and lactating women need more than their diet can supply, so supplements of 30 to 60 milligrams are recommended. The following are good dietary sources of iron:

| | |
|---|---|
| Beef liver (4 ounces) | 8.9 mgs |
| Beef pot roast (4 ounces) | 3.8 |
| Blackstrap molasses (1 tablespoon) | 3.2 |
| Spinach (1 cup, steamed) | 2.2 |
| Egg yolk (1 medium) | .94 |
| Peach (1 medium) | .6 |
| Wheat germ (1 tablespoon) | .5 |

Chelated iron supplements are more easily absorbed and less constipating than inorganic forms like ferrous sulfate. Ferrous sulfate can destroy vitamin E so if taken it should be spaced several hours apart from intake of vitamin E. Organic iron supplements (ferrous gluconate, fumerate, citrate, or peptonate) do not destroy vitamin E. Vitamin C and copper enhance iron absorption, whereas too much calcium inhibits it. By the way, cooking foods in iron skillets increases their iron content.

Taking too much iron is harmful and may cause liver damage or weakening of the bones. Excessive iron intake can result from too much iron in the water supply, excessive dietary intake, environmental exposure, or using too many iron pills.

### Chromium

Chromium, another essential trace mineral, is necessary for proper sugar metabolism and growth. Most chromium, however, is lost in the processing of foods.

If you have "yes" responses to the following questions *plus* low hair chromium levels, you *may* be suffering from a chromium deficiency.

1. Do you have hypoglycemia or diabetes?
2. Do you have gum disease?
3. Is your cholesterol level elevated?

No RDA has been set for chromium, but .05 to .2 milligrams is considered a safe and adequate dietary intake by the Food and Nutritional Board of the National Academy of Sciences. Some good dietary sources of chromium are brewer's yeast, beef liver, beef, wholewheat flour, cornmeal, chicken, and clams.

Inorganic chromium salts are poorly absorbed, so chelated chromium is the preferred form. One caution: Taking chromium supplements may cause manganese levels to drop too much.

### Manganese

Manganese is yet another essential trace mineral that is largely lost in food processing. Manganese activates enzymes necessary for proper utilization of certain vitamins. Manganese is also important in the formation of hemoglobin and and certain hormones, fat and carbohydrate synthesis, normal bone development, reproduction, and normal nervous system functioning.

With low manganese levels in hair or blood tests, positive replies to the following questions *may* indicate a manganese deficiency.

1. Do you have:
   —Gum disease?
   —Muscle and coordination problems?
   —Dizziness, ear noises, or loss of hearing?
2. Is fatigue a major symptom for you?

No RDA for manganese has been set, although an estimate of 2.5 to 5 milligrams is given. Manganese levels in foods may vary, depending on where the food is grown and in what soil, but some good dietary sources are:

| | |
|---|---|
| Rice bran (3 ounces) | 26.0 mgs[6] |
| Walnuts (3 ounces) | 15.0 |
| Spinach (3 ounces) | 15.0 to .2 |
| Wheat bran (3 ounces) | 14.0 |
| Strawberries (3 ounces) | .33 |
| Oatmeal (3 ounces) | 3.0 to .3 |
| Egg yolk (3 ounces) | .10 |

Manganese is available in multimineral preparations or as manganese citrate or gluconate tablets. Excessive manganese supplements may be harmful and may cause chromium levels to drop.

## ■ LOOKING AT YOUR ESSENTIAL FATTY ACIDS

Essential fatty acids (EFA), which result from the digestive breakdown of fats and oils, are the precursors for a powerful group of complex molecules known as prostaglandins, which control a multitude of essential functions. Sources of EFA in the diet may not be sufficient; B vitamins and certain minerals must also be present as enzyme cofactors. Researchers are now recognizing that a lack of EFA, particularly one called Omega3-EFA, is another contributing factor to allergies and many other diseases, including heart disease, arthritis, bursitis, cancer, high blood pressure, irritable bowel, multiple sclerosis, and other immune diseases.

One pioneer in this area is biochemist Donald O. Rudin, who has hypothesized that these EFA-deficiency diseases may result from our changing food supply.[7] He believes that for 50 years we have been systematically destroying trace EFA by massive chemical refining (hydrogenation) of food oils and by modern mechanical milling of grains. We have also been using certain foods and food oils (olive, corn, cottonseed, peanut, safflower, coconut, and sunflower) low in Omega3-EFA to replace oils (linseed, walnut, soybean, and chestnut) rich in this EFA. Refining foods has also depleted them of essential vitamins and minerals which function with Omega3-EFA. According to Dr. Rudin, destruction of dietary fiber is another contributing factor because lack of fiber increases the need for Omega3-EFA. High sugar consumption also interferes with the breakdown of fats into EFA. Dr. Rudin has observed that adding Omega3-EFA to the diet along with some other dietary changes has led to dramatic improvement in many patients suffering from these illnesses.

For a clue to whether you *might* be deficient in EFA, look for positive responses to the following questions.

1. Do you have scalp or eyebrow dandruff? Dry, flaky skin? Cracks in your hands, flaking eczema, or callous formations?
2. Is fatigue a major symptom for you?
3. Are you oversensitive to cold?
4. Is your alcohol tolerance poor?
5. Do you have:
   —Arthritis, bursitis, or tendonitis?
   —Glaucoma?
   —Tinnitus, or ringing in your ears?
   —Any immune disease?
   —Chronic bacterial infections?
   —Schizophrenia, manic-depressive psychosis, or phobias?

—Intestinal disorders?
—Cardiovascular disease?

Dr. Rudin suggests the following program as a corrective measure:[8]

1. Take 1 tablespoon (or 10 capsules) of food-grade linseed oil with each meal 3 times a day. *If you are drug-sensitive or have immune problems, start with 1 teaspoon per day and increment by one teaspoon per day until you reach your optimal dose.*
2. Avoid all hydrogenated oils and margarines. For cooking and salad oils, use only cold-pressed non-hydrogenated soybean, walnut, wheat germ, or linseed oils.
3. Continue linseed oil at least 2 months, dropping to a lower maintenance dose when symptoms are relieved. Otherwise increase dose to 2 tablespoons with each meal.

Caution, however, is necessary in following these guidelines. *Excessive oil may lead to recurrence of the very symptoms you are trying to relieve!* For some, just one to one and a half teaspoons will bring on symptoms. There may be a very narrow margin between a relieving dose and a toxic one, which causes symptoms to return. If you are not sure that the dose you are taking is the optimal one for you, try doubling it and then note whether your symptoms are better or worse. *Or* cut your dose in half and see if you're better or not.

The reason I strongly recommend caution with this regime is that I myself became very sick from taking several tablespoons of linseed oil a day. I couldn't figure out why my back ached so much and why I was so depressed until I contacted Dr. Rudin. He explained that one's symptoms may become much worse through taking too much linseed oil. By first reducing my dose to one teaspoon per day, and then gradually increasing it until I reached five teaspoons per day, I did find relief for my allergy symptoms. Later, I gradually reduced my dose so that I now only require one-fourth teaspoon each day. I can tell when to *decrease* my dose because my hands start to crack and my face becomes dry and scaly. Selecting one symptom, like dry skin, as a monitor makes it easier to determine when to increase or decrease the dose. If the symptom gets worse when you increase the dose, then you know you should decrease it. One additional point: Surprisingly, despite being a universal reactor, I have not had any allergy problems with the linseed oil itself. Some allergic people, however, do have trouble tolerating it and may want to try a fish oil preparation or another vegetable oil high in the Omega3-EFA.

Megadoses of most vitamins should *not* be used with this regime because there seems to be a powerful synergistic effect between some vitamins and the linseed oil. Dr. Rudin, however, does suggest that vitamin C (500 to 2,000 mgs), zinc (30 mgs), selenium (.003 mg), and vitamin E (30 to 100 IU) be used daily with the linseed oil. He also recommends using one to three tablespoons of bran or one-third that amount of psyllium seed (available in health food stores) along with yogurt (if tolerated) before meals to increase dietary fiber and encourage healthy intestinal bacteria.

Other researchers have treated similar diseases and symptoms with a different essential fatty acid (Omega6-EFA) found in evening-primrose oil and have reported good results.[9]

## ■ TAKING CARE OF DIGESTIVE DISORDERS

Nutritionally oriented physicians have observed that several kinds of digestive disorders may contribute to food and chemical sensitivities.[10] Just listen to any antacid commercial and you'll know that too much stomach acid causes indigestion. Too much stomach acid can also contribute to food allergies. But another cause of indigestion is too little stomach acid, and this, too, affects allergies. Hydrochloric acid is necessary for the complete breakdown of foods into their smallest components. If the food isn't digested completely, largely molecules of the partially digested food are absorbed into the bloodstream, where the body reacts to them as foreign invaders, generating allergic symptoms.

Impaired functioning of the pancreas may also lead to allergic problems. The pancreas produces a variety of essential digestive enzymes that break down foods in the small intestine. The pancreas is also responsible for maintaining the proper neutral to alkaline environment in the small intestine as the enzymes won't function in an acid medium.

If you answer "yes" to the following questions, you *may* be deficient in hydrochloric acid or pancreatic enzymes.

1. Did your hair analysis show low levels for many minerals?
2. Do you have excess gas, bloating, chronic constipation, or low-grade diarrhea?
3. Are you over 60? (Nutrient malabsorption increases with age.)
4. Have you experienced trouble digesting meats? Is there often undigested food in your bowel movements?

If you suspect you're low in stomach acid, your doctor may order a radiotelemetry test to measure the acid–alkaline levels (pH) in your stomach, although this is another one of those controversial tests. The test involves swallowing a plastic, enclosed, battery-operated, pH-sensitive radio transmitter. In the stomach, this device radios out to a recorder the pH of the stomach fluids. It then passes through the intestines and out of the body. A blood test for the enzymes amylase and lipase may indicate whether or not you are producing sufficient pancreatic enzymes.

If you are deficient in hydrochloric acid, supplements of betaine hydrochloride or glutamic acid hydrochloride tablets are available at most health food stores. Most doctors recommend starting with just one tablet before each meal for several days and then increasing it to two or three if no bad reaction occurs. Something's wrong if you experience heartburn, increased gas, stomach pains, or anything else unusual. Don't take any more. Baking soda in water will neutralize the reaction. Obviously, someone with a history of ulcers should *never* take hydrochloric acid. Nor should anyone taking aspirin or aspirinlike drugs take these drugs with hydrochloric acid.

Pancreatic enzymes can usually be taken safely, unless you're allergic to their sources. They are commonly derived from beef, pork, or fruits (pineapple, papaya).

# 12

# Limiting Your Exposure to Toxic Metals

Excessive exposure to heavy metals may be another underlying cause of allergies and certain physical and mental illnesses. Some people have excessive levels of several toxic metals. These metals seem to interact synergistically so that their total effect is greater than the sum of the effects of each toxic metal.

## ■ MERCURY

Problems with mercury may arise either from toxic levels in the body or a hypersensitive reaction. The body has trouble getting rid of mercury, so it may gradually accumulate. And too much mercury in the body has long been recognized as a cause of severe psychiatric and neurological symptoms. Workers who used mercury in the felt hat-manufacturing process often got the shakes and were mentally unstable, thus the expression "mad as a hatter." Today, mercury compounds are widely used in various industries that make thermometers, batteries, scientific equipment, chlorine, paper pulp, plastics, and fungicides. Burning coal also releases mercury into the atmosphere. Mercury-contaminated fish is probably the most publicized current source of mercury poisoning.[1] But mercurous compounds have been used for centuries in drugs, poisoning both patients and doctors. They can still be purchased over the counter in some antiseptics, nose sprays, cosmetics, and hemorrhoid preparations, although they must meet safety standards.

Yet another source of mercury is now recognized as a major cause of mercury poisoning—the silver amalgam fillings in your mouth! Most silver fillings contain 50% or more mercury. They are widely used because they are cheaper and easier to handle than gold. In fact, American dentists are using over 200,000 pounds of mercury annually.[2] While it's known that the amalgam material is hazardous to dentists and their technicians, it's been assumed that the fillings, once placed in the teeth, are not dangerous for the patient. Now, some observant dentists, like pioneer Hal Huggins, have measured the mercury vapor given off by fillings in the mouth and found that the amount of vapor often exceeds the safety standard set by government for industrial exposures. These dentists point out that body heat increases mercury vapors and saliva acts as an electrolyte, helping the mercury leach into the body system.[3]

Using hair, blood, and urine tests, dental researchers have reported abnormal mercury levels in individuals with silver–mercury fillings and neurological disorders. Removal of the fillings often brought dramatic relief from symptoms.[4] Interest then spread to patients with other kinds of problems. It was discovered that mercury intoxication can mimic a myriad of medical diseases and symptoms—fatigue, headaches, cardiac disorders (chest pain, angina, high blood pressure, low blood pressure, and tachycardia), emotional problems, immune system disorders (multiple sclerosis, leukemia, Hodgkins disease, lupus, and Crohn's disease), collagen diseases, and allergies! Blood counts, electrocardiograms, mercury levels, and electrical current in the mouth were monitored before and after mercury removal. As the symptoms improved or disappeared, these test results returned to normal.[5] Similar reactions to the nickel castings used in dentistry have also been observed.

Although these dentists suspect that just about everyone is sensitive to mercury to some degree, they especially want to identify people who are hypersensitive. As a preliminary check on your possible sensitivity, ask yourself the following questions. Positive answers *suggest* you may be mercury-sensitive if you have silver fillings in your teeth.

1. Did your symptoms begin or become worse during or after the placement of silver fillings?
2. When you have your teeth cleaned, are your symptoms worse?
3. Is your temperature often subnormal (96°–97° F)?
4. Do you have an amalgam tatoo (a pigmentation in the gum tissue, usually caused by the fracture of an amalgam filling during tooth extraction)?
5. Are you bothered by a metallic taste in your mouth?
6. When you chew gum, are your symptoms worse?
7. Do you often suffer from fatigue, headaches, or cold hands and feet?
8. Is your white blood count typically high or low for no obvious reason?
9. Do you have low or high blood pressure?
10. To your knowledge, have you ever reacted adversely to any medications or cosmetics containing mercury?

11. Does your work involve contact with mercury compounds?
12. Do you use a mercury-vapor sunlamp?

What else can you do to confirm your suspicions that you may be hypersensitive to mercury? A 24-hour mercury patch test is now available to your doctor or dentist to help identify the hypersensitive person.[6] A solution containing mercury chloride is placed on a bandaid on the forearm. Blood pressure, pulse, temperature, and sometimes blood counts and electrocardiograms are taken before. The patient remains in the office for an hour in case symptoms develop, as they may in the super-sensitive persons (I took only 15 minutes to react!). If symptoms develop at any time during the 24 hours, the patch is removed and the area washed well with soap and water. The test is considered positive. The patient returns 24 hours later, when the same preliminary tests (blood pressure, pulse, etc.) are again performed and any significant changes noted. Redness and swelling at the site are also indicative of a positive response.

Hair analysis may also identify the mercury-toxic patients. Hair mercury levels of .5 to .8 parts per million (ppm) reflect the average exposure in healthy people. Dr. Huggins has observed that mercury-toxic patients frequently have very low hair levels (.0 to .4 ppm), suggesting they have trouble excreting mercury from their systems. Levels above 1 ppm indicate either above-average exposure, resulting in increased levels in tissues, or that something has stimulated the person to excrete stored-up mercury at a greater-than-normal rate.[7]

Another test that helps identify mercury-toxic patients measures the electrical potential given off by their fillings. Currents may be either positive or negative. A negative current especially suggests that the patient is super-sensitive to mercury.[8] Mercury vapors can also be measured by special equipment.[9]

But before you run to your dentist to have your fillings replaced, you should consider several things. To begin with, your dentist may not believe that mercury fillings can be harmful. After all, the official word of the American Dental Association is that silver fillings are not hazardous to your health. And it probably won't be cheap to have your fillings replaced if you have a whole mouth full. Either quartz and plastic or gold are used. Quartz isn't practical for some fillings in some teeth, so gold (expensive) may be the only alternative. Although reactions to these materials are rare, they are possible. If you're highly sensitive to chemicals, there's another difficulty. You may have trouble having dental work done because of the anesthetics used. Finally, just removing the fillings may not be enough. You will probably need to use appropriate dietary supplements to help the body get rid of the mercury accumulated in the tissues. Dr. Huggins uses vitamin C, a special balanced mineral supplement, and pancreatic enzymes to increase the cell permeability so the mercury can be excreted.

If you are hypersensitive to mercury, removing the fillings may initially increase your symptoms for several days or weeks as the mercury is dumped into your system.[10] It's important to use a dentist who is aware of these side effects. Several steps can be taken to reduce the likelihood of a reaction. If you have many fillings, it's advisable to replace them a quadrant or two at a time, not all at once. Removing negatively charged fillings before positively charged ones (determined by measuring the electrical potential) also reduces the chances of a reaction. Again, supplementation with appropriate trace minerals, pancreatic enzymes, and vitamin C before and after removal reduces symptoms. Don't be surprised, however, if your symptoms flair up again 21 days after the fillings are removed. Dr. Huggins has observed that the immune system seems to have a 21-day cycle, so there may be a delayed response to the mercury-dumping. If you do experience intensified symptoms after the fillings are removed, you can console yourself (as I did) with this thought: The mercury must have been significantly contributing to my symptoms or I wouldn't be feeling so bad! And, anyhow, the reaction only lasts a few days.

Of course, there are no guarantees. You could go to all the expense and aggravation and experience no improvement in your condition.

## ■ LEAD

People today may have lead levels more than 500 times greater than those of several hundred years ago. Lead is present naturally in the earth's crust, but massive quantities have been introduced into our immediate environment through industrial use. You may be eating or drinking lead-contaminated foods or beverages, as well as breathing in lead-containing fumes from auto exhaust, and lead smelters and other industrial sources. And lead accumulates in your body; it's estimated that your body excretes less lead than is taken in.

Excessive lead can cause mental retardation in young children and hyperactivity and learning disorders in older ones. In adults, lead toxicity may generate a variety of serious neurological, emotional, and gastrointestinal disorders. Lead poisoning is apparently quite frequent in juvenile delinquents and adult criminals.[11]

Is overexposure to lead a possible cause of your

difficulties? Positive answers to the following questions *may* suggest lead poisoning.

1. Are you irritable, severely depressed, or hyperactive?
2. Do you have trouble concentrating? Is your memory poor?
3. Have you lost your appetite? Do you suffer from abdominal pain, vomiting, or constipation?
4. Are you bothered by headaches?
5. Do you often feel weak? Are you pale?
6. Do you have arthritislike symptoms?
7. Have you been exposed to old lead paint chips or dust?
8. Are you frequently exposed to leaded gas fumes, exhaust fumes, or heavy traffic? Do you jog along a busy street? Live in an area of high air pollution?
9. Is your water soft (more acidic) and do you have lead pipes?
10. Do you use:
    —Lead-glazed pottery?
    —Cosmetics, hair dyes, or hair-darkening preparations containing lead?

In addition to the kinds of lead exposure implicated in the questions, you may be taking in lead through the following: newsprint, comic books, and colored ads; toothpaste tubes and soft metal containers; lead-contaminated bonemeal or dolomite; and cigarette smoke and ashes.

If you suspect lead toxicity, see your doctor for a lead blood and hair analysis.

## ■ ALUMINUM

Although aluminum is plentiful in the earth's surface, only low concentrations are found in plants and animals, and there is no conclusive evidence that aluminum is essential for human life. When you think of aluminum, you probably think of aluminum foil and cookware. You may not be aware of other ways your body daily comes in contact with aluminum—through antacids, deodorants, polluted water, some toothpastes, food additives, and baking powder. Whether or not these sources increase body levels of aluminum is, however, controversial.

Some doctors do report physical and mental symptoms caused by too much aluminum in the body.[12] Specifically, they describe gastrointestinal irritation, poor concentration, poor memory, and irritability. High aluminum levels are often found in patients with other kinds of toxic metal poisoning. You *may* be getting too much aluminum if you find yourself answering "yes" to the following questions.

1. Do you suffer from mental disturbances?
2. Are you troubled by nausea and constipation?
3. Is fatigue a major symptom?
4. Do you suffer from loss of appetite?
5. Is excessive perspiration a problem?
6. Do you use aluminum cookware or coffee pots?
7. Does your water contain too much aluminum?
8. Do you use antacids, deodorants, or baking powder that contain aluminum compounds?

If you suspect aluminum toxicity, see your doctor for an aluminum blood and hair analysis.

## ■ OTHER METALS

Cadmium is another heavy metal that can cause serious problems if body levels are excessive. Loss of appetite or sense of smell and damage to the heart, blood vessels, brain, and kidneys have been reported.[13]

Environmental sources of cadmium exposure include cigarette smoke, contaminated drinking water, industrial dusts, galvanized pipes, paints, welding, and zinc smelters.

Copper may also present difficulties, although—unlike mercury, lead, aluminum, and cadmium—it is an essential trace metal involved in bone formation, healing, red blood cell formation, cognitive processes, and emotional states. Too little copper can cause copper-deficiency anemia, bone changes, alterations in hair color and texture, weakness, impaired respiration, and skin sores. But copper deficiencies are rare since copper is found in many foods. Copper poisoning, on the other hand, is more common, causing insomnia, irritability, and other emotional problems.[14] Toxic copper levels may stem from use of copper water pipes or copper cookware, a low zinc level, or excessive intake, either in the diet or through copper supplements.

Like copper, nickel, cobalt, and tin are present as trace elements in our bodies, playing a role in our metabolism. Nevertheless, in excessive amounts they are toxic.

# 13

# Reducing Stress in Your Day-to-Day Life

Stress can make allergies worse, and it may trigger reactions by altering body chemistry. Anxiety or tension over everyday concerns isn't the only common source of stress. Infections, lack of sleep, and exposure to cold or heat also create stress. Reducing stress in your life should improve your overall allergic condition.

## RELIEF THROUGH EXERCISE

Not only does exercise help reduce stress, but it also helps relieve allergy symptoms by helping the body get rid of excess water and toxins. Choose some form of exercise that "turns you on," then stick with it. My husband and I took up bicycling last summer and were surprised by how much we enjoyed it and how much better we felt. We were sorry to have cold weather arrive. Exercising with a friend or a group may be more fun than doing it alone. And it may keep you at it.

Still, some precautions are necessary. Not every form of exercise is good for everybody. If you're not used to exercise, consult your doctor about the type of exercise and the duration that's best for *you.* Always start slowly. Also, be sure to choose exercise that is compatible with your allergies. For example, excessive exertion may trigger attacks in asthmatics. Cold air or water may precipitate hives and wheezing to some allergic people. Hay fever victims may be uncomfortable swimming. And although chemically sensitive people may enjoy swimming in lakes, they may need to avoid chlorinated pools.

## ■ LEARNING TO RELAX

There are really three aspects to relaxation—reducing thought processes, slowing down physiological processes, and decreasing muscular tension. One of these may be more important for you than the others. Moreover, many relaxation techniques are available. If you have severe trouble relaxing, finding an expert (psychologist, psychiatrist, rehabilitation therapist, or muscle therapist) trained in relaxation techniques might well be worth the time and expense.

Here's one method for muscle relaxation I've found helpful, especially when you're starting out. Basically, it involves deliberately tensing each muscle as much as possible and then relaxing that muscle. In this way you can perceive how tense muscles feel and how good it feels to relax them

1. Find a comfortable couch, bed, or recliner that supports your whole body. Choose a quiet, dimly lit private room.
2. Begin by tensing your fists for 6 to 10 seconds. Then let go and enjoy how relaxed they feel for 40 seconds or so.
3. Proceed with your upper arms. Pull up with your

fists clenched, then press down with your palms flat. Always relax in between tensings.

4. Next work on your face and head. Wrinkle your forehead as though worried. Then wrinkle it as though angry. Close your eyes tightly while making the angry look. To tense lips, purse them tightly together. For your jaw, clench your teeth together. Finally, press your tongue tightly against the roof of your mouth.
5. Move on to your neck, shoulders, and back. Tense your neck by pressing your head back hard against the surface of the couch (or whatever). Then roll your head slowly to the right, to the left, back to the middle, then down to your chest. Now relax. Tense your shoulders and upper back by shrugging your shoulders up high. After relaxing, arch your lower back.
6. To work on your chest and abdomen, start by breathing in deeply and holding your breath as long as possible. Tense your abdomen by pulling in your stomach muscles to look skinny. Then tense your muscles as if someone were going to hit you in the middle.
7. Finally, tense your buttocks and legs by first pressing your legs down hard against the surface. Next point toes downward like a ballet dancer. Then point your toes upwards, toward your head.
8. Throughout the exercises, breathe deeply and slowly. Occasionally take deeper breaths and notice how good you feel when you release the air.

Another method you might try to feel more relaxed and to relieve pain in specific areas is foot reflexology. You can either do it to yourself or have someone else massage your feet. The idea is to knead all areas of the top and bottom of the foot, including the toes. If you find an especially tender area that spot should receive extra attention, the equivalent spot on the other foot should also be massaged. You may be surprised how tender certain areas are. Experts in foot reflexology claim that there are specific points in the feet that correspond with the health of various parts of the body.[1] For example, a headache may be relieved by massaging, in a circular motion, a small area on the inside underside of the big toe. There are also equivalent spots on the hands that may be massaged similarly when it's not practical to rub your feet.

One other method of learning relaxation I'd recommend is biofeedback. In one kind of biofeedback, electrodes are placed over tense muscles. The biofeedback machine responds by making a noise whose frequency varies, depending on how tense the muscle is. By listening to the noise, you can learn what it feels like to be more and more relaxed. Biofeedback techniques have been most beneficial in helping patients with headaches, muscle aches, asthma, and high blood pressure learn to relax, and thus reduce or eliminate their symptoms. Check with your local hospital, university, or mental health facility to see if biofeedback therapy is available in your area.

## ■ COMING TO TERMS WITH THE STRESS OF HAVING ALLERGIES

Allergic people have the same everyday stresses and psychological problems that other people have. But on top of these problems they must cope with their allergic reactions, which are stressful in themselves.

First of all, there's the stress of undiagnosed allergies. What if you're not feeling well, but no one seems to know what's wrong? You may wonder: "Is it all in my head? My doctor can't find anything wrong. Maybe I'm just imagining all this." Some doctors may encourage this self-doubt. When the lab tests they have taken are normal, they declare nothing is physically wrong. They may then prescribe tranquilizers or refer you to a psychiatrist. Nor are family and friends always understanding. They, too, may express disbelief about the "realness" of your symptoms. All of this just compounds the problem.

And if you don't know why you're feeling so bad, you may well feel scared and panicky. Maybe you have some terrible degenerative disease. If most of your symptoms are mental, you may fear you're losing your mind. Once you learn that allergy is the cause of your problems, at least you know what you're dealing with. When you're feeling awful, you can remind yourself that the reaction *will* pass and you *will* feel better.

Even beyond your natural fears and self-doubts, there may be a problem. Allergic bodies tend to react to an allergen with edema—extra water in all the tissues. The brain may be waterlogged too, causing depression and anxiety. So your perception of yourself and your relationship to others may be distorted. Everything may seem hopeless during a bad reaction, although the same problems seem manageable or nonexistent when the reaction subsides. If you're experiencing a bad reaction, hang in there and remember that you will feel better. With experience, you may be able to learn to tell the difference between a depression caused by a "real" problem and one caused by an allergic reaction. As a start, ask yourself if there's a legitimate psychological reason for your depression. If there isn't, ask yourself what you've just eaten or been exposed to that might be causing your depression.

Fatigue is another unwelcome problem during a reaction. This fatigue isn't just the normal tiredness you get from working all day. It's feeling exhausted and drained. You may feel so tired you can hardly get out of bed and put one foot in front of the other. Following your normal routine seems impossible. You may be so tired both mentally and physically that you can't even remember which medicine to take or recall what you've been exposed to. Sleep helps some people, but for others it seems to make the fatigue worse. As hard as it may be, try exercising—it may help by hastening the excretion of the chemicals causing the problems and the extra water. Increased oxygen also helps. Breathe deeply.

How you handle your allergies depends on your personality. Different people respond differently. At first, you may deny your condition: "Allergies are for other people, not for me. If I ignore it, it'll go away. Bring on the cake and ice cream, and don't forget the chocolate topping!" This approach may work for awhile, but it's not likely to last.

My own response has been to seek as much information as possible. I gain comfort in understanding and learning as much as I can. I feel more in control of my allergies that way. And it's an optimistic approach. I'm always searching for newer and better answers because I refuse to believe that my family will always have our allergies. We're already so much better. The goal is total recovery.

Sharing your knowledge and experience with others is another way to cope with your situation. In helping form an allergy support group, I had the chance to talk with others in the same boat. What I've gained is valuable information, as well as new friends. If your city doesn't have such a group, start one yourself! All you need is a few allergy victims and your group will soon grow. One way to get started is to write a letter to the "action line" of your local newspaper, inquiring if such an organization exists and giving your phone number so interested readers can call you. For speakers, draw on the talent in your community: a psychologist to talk about and demonstrate relaxation techniques, a nutritionist or dietician to talk about food values, a family counselor to discuss ways to deal with stress in the home. Our electric company demonstrated ways to cook without some of the common allergy-causing foods while throwing in tips on energy-saving techniques. You can share recipes, tapes, books, and local food sources. What doctors seem to be helping their patients the most and are open to new ideas? Are any local dentists trained in balancing body chemistry? Most important is that you'll find people who have the same feelings, frustrations, and problems you've been struggling with.

All of this is helpful. But what about the allergy problem itself? Being allergic is often expensive. You may need a special diet of expensive foods. Your house may need alterations. You may have to change the kinds of clothes you wear. Medical bills may be out of sight. Some insurance companies have tried to deny payment for certain procedures like provocative testing and neutralization therapy, although some patients have successfully sued them for reimbursement. It's all more stress!

And allergies are time-consuming. Someone has to shop for the foods allowed on the diet. Several different meals may have to be prepared if different family members have different allergies. Someone has to keep the house clean and allergy-free.

Another frustration is having your behavior restricted. You may not be able to do what everyone else does. You may not be able to eat the same foods. Perfume and smoke may keep you from group situations. Traveling may be difficult.

The biggest frustration of all may be that other people don't believe you. Your doctor may dismiss you as a hypochondriac. At least one close relative is bound to declare it's all in your head. Friends may consider your restrictions ridiculous. Since *they've* never heard of such a thing, then such reactions can't occur.

How do you cope with these nonbelievers? If your doctor isn't helpful, find one who is knowledgeable and supportive. For friends, you might try to educate them. Give them books to read; invite them to go with you to an allergy meeting. But if that fails, don't fret about it. Believe in the knowledge you have gained. And be assertive if something they're doing (smoking or wearing perfume) is making you sick.

Still, all these frustrations add stress. There isn't a magical solution. Receiving professional counseling from a minister, social worker, psychologist, or psychiatrist may be quite helpful, especially if severe depression is involved. It's important, though, to find the right person—someone who understands the relationship between allergy and behavior and is supportive of other treatment methods you're using. A counselor who is coping well with his or her own allergies is ideal!

For some of the everyday problems that come up around allergies, especially food sensitivities, I can offer a few tips from my own experience. These suggestions may help you to add your own.

### Trying Not to Cheat on Your Diet

If you find it difficult to stay on your diet, welcome to the club! Let's face it, we all cheat from time to time. The addictive nature of food allergy itself makes it hard not to cheat. Sometimes you can cheat and not experience symptoms. But the next time you may really make yourself sick. Often it's hard to predict how you'll react. Here are a few pointers that may help you stick to your diet.

1. Think about how bad you feel when you break your diet. Is it worth feeling that bad? Admittedly, sometimes the answer is "yes"! But don't you feel *better* on your diet?
2. Remember: The longer you stay away from craved foods, the easier it should be to avoid them. I find I don't want sugar if I avoid it completely. Once I start cheating, then my sugar cravings return, and they're hard to deny. One birthday I had a small piece of cake with my family, took the leftover cake to the kitchen and ate all the icing. You can imagine the rest of the story!
3. Substitute some other food you do enjoy that doesn't make you sick. If everyone else is eating birthday cake, have a slice of allowed homemade pumpkin or zucchini bread.
4. When you experience cravings, try drinking lots of water. Go for a walk or exercise. Take a bath.
5. Keep problem foods out of the house altogether, or store them in your most inaccessible closet. Make it hard to satisfy your cravings.
6. Don't go to the grocery store on an empty stomach or when your resistance is low. If I shop first thing in the morning, I don't even consider buying what I shouldn't eat. By late afternoon, when I'm tired and hungry, my willpower disappears. Make a list before you go and stick to it.
7. Always carry a safe snack food with you. On a coffee break at work, eat these snacks. Sit as far from the vending machines as you can.
8. Reward yourself for your willpower. If you resist buying those luscious, sugary donuts, put that money aside to buy something special for yourself.

9. Don't cheat before some important event. If you have to speak to the PTA, take an important exam, or negotiate a difficult business deal, walk the straight and narrow before. Then be sure to reward yourself afterward for a job well done and for your strong willpower.

Still, we all have times when we deliberately break our diets. Perhaps these suggestions will help you survive.

1. Make sure whatever you eat, you enjoy it so much that it's worth the price you pay. At least when you're feeling awful you can say it was really worth it. Nothing is worse than being violently ill on something that you didn't enjoy.
2. If possible, schedule your cheating on a weekend when you'll have the next day to recuperate. If my family goes out to eat, it's usually on a Friday night. Although we won't feel great Saturday, we will feel better Sunday and be in good shape for school and work on Monday.
3. Try to restrict your cheating to one day a week. It's probably better to blow it one day than to spread your cheating over several days.
4. If you know you're going to cheat in a few days, be extra good in the meantime. Give your body a chance to fight the food you're going to eat. After a "binge," allow yourself extra rest and sleep.
5. Be sure to take any medicine your doctor might prescribe. Some medicines can be taken before you indulge; others afterward. I take an antihistamine and extra vitamins before I go out to eat.
6. Choose your poisons carefully. If you're going to buy a cake, you don't have to choose the junkiest. Some baked goods are an improvement over others.

7. If you're like my family and can't stop eating anything sweet once you start, try dividing up your special treat. What we do is to allow ourselves only one piece each. Before we eat a bite we give the rest away to neighbors or even put it down the disposal! Wasteful? Yes! Shameful? Maybe. But we save ourselves from becoming violently ill.
8. Don't feel guilty. Guilt feelings are a waste of time and energy you don't have. If you react to what you've just eaten, you may be tempted to ask yourself how you could be so stupid and weak! Don't vow to never cheat again because that's probably an impossible goal. Just try to do better.

### Coping with Eating Out

If you're like most Americans, you probably eat several meals a week away from home. Allergies and restaurants often don't mix very well. Not only is the food a problem, but the chemically sensitive person may be bothered by cigarette smoke, restroom deodorants, candles, or a gas stove. Here are some suggestions so you won't have to forgo all the pleasures of eating out, even if you're severely allergic.

1. Keep a list of restaurants where you seem to do pretty well. Include what you ordered from their menus.
2. If you're familiar with the restaurant, try to decide before you go what you will order. Then stick to your plan.
3. Avoid fast-food restaurants, as they are usually a disaster for the allergic person sensitive to wheat, sugar, additives, beef, or milk.
4. Look for a restaurant with a salad bar, where you can build a salad with safe vegetables. If necessary, bring a small container of salad dressing you tolerate.

5. Avoid alcohol. Instead, order sparkling water with a twist of lime.
6. If you have trouble resisting all the goodies you should avoid, try eating a satisfying snack before you go. Keeping your blood sugar normal should help you make a rational decision.
7. If sugar is a problem, avoid dessert or order fresh fruit, if available. Reward yourself with something safe and tasty when you get home.
8. If you know the retaurant supplies a basket of irresistible rolls, ask for only a certain number or none at all.
9. Be sure to carry any medication or vitamins with you at all times in case you have a reaction.

What about dining at a friend's home?

1. Call your hostess before you go and ask what's being served. If it is off your diet and would cause you misery, ask if you may bring something for yourself.
2. Don't trust your eyes. Ask your hostess what a certain casserole contains. My mother, who is very chocolate-sensitive, became ill after eating chili at a dinner party. Only later did she learn that chocolate was one of the "special" ingredients. Of course her allergies to tomatoes and onions didn't help!
3. Don't give long speeches and explanations when you turn down a food. Simply say, "No, thank you. I don't care for any." If pushed for a reason, explain very briefly that the food causes a physical reaction that anyone can relate to—like a headache—but don't say it makes you depressed or spacey. They may not understand.

### Finding a Way to Entertain

If you're doing the entertaining, then you have more control over the environment and menu, but you're bound to encounter some problems.

1. If you're chemically sensitive, be aware that some guests may arrive drenched in perfume or aftershave and then proceed to smoke like chimneys. You want your guests to have a relaxed, happy time, but you don't want to end up sick or have your house contaminated with the chemicals. Close friends will already know and understand your problem, but new acquaintances won't. Be assertive. Explain when you invite new guests that smoking and perfumes make you sick and you would appreciate their consideration. Don't supply ashtrays. Keep windows and doors open a little for ventilation. Run your air cooler.
2. Avoid alcohol yourself. No one will notice or care if you are drinking something else.
3. For your menu, choose foods you can eat or ones you can discreetly avoid without anyone noticing. But be sure to have enough safe foods so you won't be tempted.
4. Have an allowed snack before the party to keep your blood sugar up.

Final acceptance of your problems is important. Learn what your allergens are, how to limit exposures, what underlying factors cause your allergies and what you can do about them, and how you can relieve your symptoms if a reaction occurs. Keep looking for better answers, but go on with your life!

# SECTION FOUR

# Adapting Recipes for Elimination Diets

The following recipes should help you prepare meals while you're trying any common elimination diet. The recipes also are intended to guide and inspire you to adapt your own favorite recipes to your particular food restrictions. After all, maintaining your improved health will depend largely on whether you can learn to live happily within your limitations. You will probably find that you can still enjoy many of your favorite foods even though they're prepared slightly differently. You also may discover new foods and recipes that you've never bothered to try before.

The recipes in the following chapters are sugar-free, chocolate-free, and use ingredients without artificial colors and flavors. The recipes avoid when possible the common allergy-causing foods—milk, egg, corn, wheat, rye, and citrus. Under the title of each recipe is a list of these common foods that the recipe does *not* contain. For instance, this list may state, "No milk, egg, corn, wheat, rye, or citrus" and you know that you can safely use that recipe when you're trying the Common Foods Elimination Diet. In some recipes where alternative ingredients are listed such as "egg or egg replacer," the recipe is still listed as "no egg" since it can be prepared without eggs.

Whenever possible, the recipes use nutritious ingredients. For instance, carrots or pumpkin are added to cookies, cakes, breads, and ice cream for extra nutrition. If wheat is tolerated, wheat germ can enrich many recipes. Nuts used in cookies, breads, and cakes provide extra protein, minerals, and vitamins. Only small amounts of sweeteners are used. Instead, naturally sweet fruits are substituted.

Be adventuresome! Most recipes are easily adapted to your particular diet. You will find that you *can* enjoy both good health and delicious meals without spending hours in the kitchen.

# 14

# Making Your Own Staples

You may be able to find some of these staples without sugar, dyes, and preservatives in your supermarket or health foods store. If not, here are some easy recipes.

**UNCOLORED BUTTER**
(No egg, corn, wheat, rye, or citrus)
Makes 1 cup

*1½ pints pure whipping cream, chilled*
*1 teaspoon salt*

Using an electric mixer on high speed, beat the chilled cream until it begins to look like cornmeal mush. Continue beating until lumps are corn-kernel size.

Drain off the liquid. Run very cold water over the remaining butter and press with a wooden spoon, squeezing out and discarding the liquid. Repeat this procedure until the liquid is completely gone. Add salt and mix thoroughly. Pack into containers and refrigerate.

**WHITE SAUCE**
(No milk, egg, corn, wheat, rye, or citrus)
Makes 1 cup

*1 tablespoon pure allowed vegetable oil or uncolored butter or allowed margarine, melted*
*1 tablespoon unbleacher flour, rice flour, or potato starch flour*
*½ teaspoon salt*
*Dash of pepper*
*1 cup milk or Chicken Stock (see page 209)*

Blend shortening with flour and seasonings in a heavy saucepan. Add liquid gradually. Cook quickly, stirring constantly, until mixture thickens and bubbles.

A thicker sauce may be made by doubling the shortening and thickener used.

**MAYONNAISE**
(No milk, corn, wheat, rye, or citrus)
Makes about 14 ounces

*1 egg*
*1 teaspoon salt*
*1 teaspoon dry mustard*
*⅛ teaspoon pepper*
*1¼ cups pure allowed vegetable oil*
*3 tablespoons allowed vinegar or pure lemon juice*

Blend together egg, salt, mustard, pepper, and ¼ cup oil in a blender on high speed. With the blender still running, add an additional ½ cup oil very slowly. Then add vinegar or lemon juice. Blend in remaining ½ cup oil very slowly until mayonnaise is thick. Refrigerate in a covered glass container.

### TOMATO CATSUP

(No milk, egg, corn, wheat, rye, or citrus)
Makes about 2 cups

*½ cup allowed vinegar*
*½ teaspoon whole cloves*
*1 2-inch stick cinnamon*
*½ teaspoon celery seed*
*4 pounds (about 12 medium) tomatoes, washed and quartered*
*¼ cup water*
*2 tablespoons dried minced onion or ½ onion, finely chopped*
*⅛ teaspoon black pepper*
*¼ cup honey*
*2 teaspoons salt*

Combine vinegar, cloves, cinnamon, and celery seed in a small covered saucepan. Bring to a boil. Remove from heat. Let stand.

In a large kettle cook tomatoes, water, onion, and pepper over medium heat until tomatoes are quite soft. Put tomato mixture through sieve or food mill. Return juice to stove. Add honey and salt. Bring to a boil. Reduce heat and simmer until volume has been reduced by half. Strain vinegar into tomato mixture, discarding spices. Continue simmering until desired consistency is reached, stirring frequently. Cool and refrigerate in a covered glass container.

### MUSTARD

(No milk, corn, wheat, rye, or citrus)
Makes 2 cups

*1 cup allowed vinegar*
*1 cup dry mustard*
*2 eggs*
*½ cup honey*

Add vinegar to dry mustard and stir until lumps disappear. Cover and let sit overnight.

Pour mustard mixture into the top of a double boiler. Beat eggs. Add honey to eggs and mix. Slowly stir the egg and honey mixture into the mustard. Cook over boiling water for about 12 minutes until thickened, stirring to avoid lumps. Pour into a covered glass container and refrigerate. If this mustard is too hot for your taste, mix it with some mayonnaise.

### FRENCH DRESSING

(No milk, egg, corn, wheat, rye, or citrus)
Makes 1½ cups

*3 tablespoons honey*
*2 teaspoons salt*
*½ teaspoon pepper*
*1 teaspoon paprika*
*½ cup allowed vinegar*
*1 cup pure allowed vegetable oil*

Combine all ingredients in a covered jar. Shake thoroughly. Refrigerate. Shake well before using.

### SLAW DRESSING

(No milk, egg, corn, wheat, rye, or citrus)
Makes about 1 cup

*1 cup Mayonnaise (see page 202) or Egg-Free Mayonnaise (see page 246)*
*1 tablespoon pure lemon juice or unsweetened pineapple juice*
*4 teaspoons honey (2 teaspoons if using pineapple juice)*

Mix together thoroughly. Refrigerate in a covered jar.

## FRUIT SALAD DRESSING

(No milk, egg, corn, wheat, rye, or citrus)
Makes 1¾ cups

*1 heaping teaspoon paprika*
*½ teaspoon dry mustard*
*¼ teaspoon onion salt*
*½ teaspoon celery seed*
*1 cup pure allowed vegetable oil*
*½ cup allowed vinegar*
*⅓ cup honey*

Mix all ingredients together. Beat until well blended. Refrigerate in a covered jar for 24 hours before using.

## THOUSAND ISLAND DRESSING

(No milk, corn, wheat, rye, or citrus)
Makes 1½ cups

*1 cup Mayonnaise (see page 202)*
*¼ cup Tomato Catsup (see page 203), Tomato-Free Catsup I (see page 288), or Tomato-Free Catsup II (see page 288)*
*2 hard-cooked eggs, chopped*
*2 tablespoons capers or chopped Sweet Pickles (see page 206)*
*2 tablespoons chopped celery*
*1 teaspoon instant minced onion*

Combine all ingredients. Keep refrigerated in a covered container.

## DILL PICKLES

(No milk, egg, corn, wheat, rye, or citrus)
Makes 4 pints

*2 quarts plus 2 cups water*
*½ cup plus 2 tablespoons pickling salt*

*8 cups long strips unwaxed cucumbers or zucchini*
*2 cups allowed vinegar*
*6 cloves garlic*
*8 tablespoons dill seed*
*4 teaspoons mustard seed*

In a large bowl combine 2 quarts water and ½ cup pickling salt Place cucumber or zucchini strips in this brine and allow to soak overnight. Then rinse strips in clear cold water.

In a saucepan combine vinegar, 2 cups water, remaining 2 tablespoons pickling salt, and garlic cloves. Bring to a boil. Remove from heat and allow to steep for about 15 minutes. Meanwhile, pack the strips tightly in pint jars. In each jar, put 2 tablespoons dill seed and 1 teaspoon mustard seed. Remove the garlic from the vinegar mixture and pour while hot over the strips, making sure they are completely covered. Cool and refrigerate.

**SWEET PICKLES**
(No milk, egg, corn, wheat, rye, or citrus)
Makes 4 pints

*8 cups sliced unwaxed cucumbers or zucchini*
*5 cups water*
*¼ cup pickling salt*
*2 cups pure maple syrup*
*3 cups allowed vinegar*
*1 2-inch stick cinnamon*
*1 whole nutmeg, cracked into large pieces*
*1 teaspoon celery seed*
*1 teaspoon salt*

Soak sliced cucumber or zucchini in 4 cups water mixed with the pickling salt overnight. Then drain, rinse several times in clear water, and let stand in cold water for 3 hours. Combine the remaining ingredients with 1 cup water and bring to a boil. Pour the hot syrup over the drained slices and allow to stand overnight. Remove cinnamon stick and nutmeg. Pack into glass jars. Refrigerate.

### DRY BREAD CRUMBS

(No milk, egg, corn, wheat, rye, or citrus)

*Several slices stale allowed bread*

Preheat oven to 300°F

Place stale bread on a cookie sheet and heat until dried. Put through a blender or food processor. Store crumbs in a covered container in the refrigerator.

### SOFT BREAD CRUMBS

(No milk, egg, corn, wheat, rye, or citrus)

*Several slices stale allowed bread*

Break bread apart very lightly with your fingers.

### CROUTONS

(No milk, egg, corn, wheat, rye, or citrus)
Makes 4 cups

*4 cups allowed bread*
*2 teaspoons Italian herb seasoning*
*½ teaspoon garlic salt*
*½ cup uncolored butter or allowed margarine*

Preheat oven to 350°F

Cut bread into ½-inch cubes. Place cubes in a large baking dish and bake in oven until cubes begin to dry, about 10 minutes. Sprinkle herb seasoning and garlic salt evenly over the cubes. Drizzle with melted butter or margarine and toss to coat all cubes. Return to oven for 30 to 45 minutes, stirring every 10 minutes until croutons are very crisp and dry. Cool thoroughly. Refrigerate in a covered container.

### BREAD STUFFING

(No milk, egg, corn, wheat, rye, or citrus)
Makes enough stuffing for 10-pound turkey

*1½ teaspoons poultry seasoning*
*¼ cup nutmeg*
*2 teaspoons salt*
*8 cups Soft Bread Crumbs (see page 207)*
*2 tablespoons grated onion*
*2 eggs, slightly beaten (optional)*
*½ cup pure allowed vegetable oil*

Combine dry ingredients with bread pieces. Add onion, eggs, and oil. Mix well.

### BEEF STOCK

(No milk, egg, corn, wheat, rye, or citrus)
Makes 1 quart

*6 pounds soup bones* or *2 pounds cheap cut of beef*
*2½ quarts cold water*
*1 cup sliced onions*
*½ cup chopped celery with leaves*
*1 bay leaf*
*Several sprigs fresh parsley or dried flakes*
*2 teaspoons salt*
*Pepper, as desired*

In a large pot, cover beef bones or beef with cold water. Bring to a boil, add rest of ingredients, and simmer covered for 2 hours. Strain. Remove meat from bones and store in refrigerator for later use. Refrigerate broth. When ready to use, skim off fat and reheat.

## CHICKEN STOCK

(No milk, egg, corn, wheat, rye, or citrus)
Makes 2 quarts

*4 pounds chicken bones or whole carcass, broken up*
*4 quarts cold water*
*1 medium onion, diced, or ¼ cup instant minced onion*
*1 carrot, diced*
*Several stalks celery, diced*
*Salt and pepper to taste*

Cover chicken bones or carcass with cold water in a large pot. Add onion, carrot, and celery and bring slowly to a boil. Simmer for 2 to 3 hours. Strain, season, and cool. Refrigerate. Skim off fat on top when ready to use stock.

## SAUSAGE PATTIES

(No milk, egg, corn, wheat, rye, or citrus)
Makes 12 patties

*2 pounds coarsely ground pork or lean ground beef*
*4 teaspoons sage*
*½ teaspoon thyme*
*½ teaspoon marjoram*
*½ teaspoon basil*
*1½ teaspoons salt*
*½ teaspoon black pepper*
*⅔ cup water*
*1 tablespoon pure allowed vegetable oil*

Combine all ingredients in a large mixing bowl. Mix thoroughly. Shape into twelve patties and fry (see below), or place on a cookie sheet and freeze until firm. Package for freezing and use patties as needed.

To cook, place fresh or frozen patty in a skillet and

fry slowly in oil until fully cooked and slightly browned.

### CORN-FREE BAKING POWDER

(No milk, egg, corn, wheat, rye, or citrus)
Makes ¾ cup

*¼ cup baking soda*
*¼ cup cream of tartar*
*¼ cup potato starch*

Sift each ingredient before measuring. Mix together thoroughly. Sift again. Store baking powder in a tightly covered jar. To check if baking powder is still active, add several drops of water to a little baking powder. If it bubbles vigorously, it is still good. Use as you would any commercial double-acting baking powder.

### WHEAT PIECRUST

(No milk, egg, corn, rye, or citrus)
Makes 1 8- or 9-inch piecrust

*1 cup unbleached flour*
*2 tablespoons toasted wheat germ*
*¾ teaspoons salt*
*⅓ cup pure allowed vegetable oil*
*2 tablespoons cold milk or ice cold water*

Preheat oven to 450°F

Mix flour, wheat germ, and salt together. Measure oil and liquid into a cup, but do not mix together. Add to the flour mixture. Stir until well mixed. With your hands form the dough into a smooth ball. Place on a sheet of waxed paper and flatten a little. Cover with another sheet of waxed paper and roll out with a rolling pin to desired size and thickness. Peel off top paper. Turn over into pie pan so remaining paper is on top.

Carefully peel off paper. Fit into pan and press dough around edges. If baking only the crust, prick in several spots with a fork. Bake for 10 to 12 minutes, or until lightly browned. Double recipe for a two-crust pie.

**PIZZA CRUST**

(No milk, egg, corn, rye or citrus)
Makes 2 12-inch crusts or 3 9-inch crusts

*1 package dry yeast or 1 cake compressed yeast*
*1½ cups warm water*
*3 to 3½ cups unbleached flour or 2 cups wholewheat flour and ¾ to 1 cup unbleached flour*
*1 teaspoon salt*
*1 tablespoon pure allowed vegetable oil*

Dissolve yeast in warm water. Stir in about half the flour. Add salt. Beat well with an electric mixer for 2 to 3 minutes. Add oil. Using fingertips, work in enough remaining flour so that dough is no longer sticky. On a floured surface, knead dough for 5 to 8 minutes.

Place in a lightly greased bowl, turning dough to grease the top too. Cover with a damp cloth and let rise in a warm place until double in bulk, about 1 hour. Punch down. Divide dough into desired number of pieces. Roll each piece into a circle. Place on oiled pizza pans or in cake pans. Turn up the edges. Fill and proceed as in desired pizza recipe.

# 15

# Cooking Without Sugar

## SUGAR SUBSTITUTES

Omit sugar in appropriate recipes.

Substitute ⅓ to ½ cup honey or pure maple syrup for each cup sugar. Decrease liquids by ⅛ to ¼ cup.

Substitute ½ to ⅔ cup fructose for each cup sugar. Fructose should be avoided by those sensitive to corn. Some other individuals may not tolerate fructose either.

Substitute ½ cup date sugar for each cup sugar.

Substitute ½ cup barley malt syrup for each cup of molasses.

Substitute 1 packet Equal for 2 teaspoons sugar.

Substitute finely ground unsweetened coconut for confectioners' sugar in appropriate recipes. For example, roll donuts in coconut instead of powdered sugar.

Use naturally sweet juices or concentrated juices such as apple, grape, orange, and pineapple to add sweetness without adding sugar.

Use naturally sweet fruits like bananas, raisins, dates, pineapple, and oranges for extra sweetness while reducing or omitting sugar.

So you're sensitive to cane and beet sugars and you feel like you've kissed your last treat good-bye forever: no more cakes, pies, jams, or candy. But you *can* have these treats and others by learning to adapt your favorite recipes. Here are some tips and examples.

Some recipes call for very small amounts of sugar, a tablespoon or so. Just omit it. For example, some spaghetti recipes use a little sugar. Who needs sugar in spaghetti sauce?

**TOMATO SPAGHETTI SAUCE**
(No milk, egg, corn, wheat, rye, or citrus)
Makes 8 cups

*1½ pounds lean ground beef*
*3 cloves garlic, minced*
*1 large onion, minced*
*1 1-pound, 12-ounce can whole tomatoes, undrained and slightly chopped*
*2 6-ounce cans tomato paste*
*1½ teaspoons oregano*
*1 teaspoon dried sweet basil*
*½ teaspoon thyme*
*1 bay leaf*
*1 teaspoon salt*
*¼ teaspoon pepper*
*1 cup water*
*2 4-ounce cans chopped mushrooms, drained (optional)*

Brown the ground beef in a large saucepan. Add garlic and onion and cook slightly. Add all other ingredients and bring to a boil. Cover, reduce heat, and simmer for approximately 1 hour. Add more water if necessary.

Use immediately or store in freezer for future use.

**WHEAT BREAD OR ROLLS**

(No milk, egg, corn, rye, or citrus)

Bread recipes always call for some sugar to help the yeast grow, which makes the bread rise. Your bread will rise just fine without sugar although it may take a little longer. Or you can substitute a little honey.

Makes 2 loaves or 32 rolls

*2 packages dry yeast or 2 cakes compressed yeast*
*2 cups warm water or milk*
*1 tablespoon honey (optional)*
*2 teaspoons salt*
*¼ cup pure allowed vegetable oil*
*½ cup toasted wheat germ*
*4½ to 5 cups unbleached flour*

Preheat oven to 400°F

Dissolve yeast in warm liquid. Add honey, salt, and oil. Stir in wheat germ. Add half the flour and beat with an electric mixer on medium speed for 2 minutes. Using fingertips, slowly work in enough flour so that dough is no longer sticky. Place on floured surface and knead until dough is smooth and elastic, about 8 to 10 minutes.

For bread, place dough in a greased bowl, turning to grease the top too. Cover. Let rise in a warm place until double in bulk, about 1 or 2 hours. Punch dough down. Let dough rise again until double in bulk, about 1 hour. Punch down. Place on lightly floured surface.

For bread, divide dough into two parts. Make into two loaves and place in two greased 8½ × 4½-inch loaf pans. Cover and let rise until double in bulk, about ½ hour. Bake for 25 to 30 minutes. Remove from pans. If bottom of loaf sounds hollw when tapped, bread is done. Cool on wire racks.

For rolls, place two 1-inch balls in greased muffin pans. Brush with allowed oil or melted butter. Cover. Let rolls rise till double in bulk, about ½ hour. Bake for 12 to 15 minutes.

**BUBBLE COFFEE CAKE**

(No milk, egg, corn, rye, or citrus)

For special occasions, this dough is sweetened with honey or pure maple syrup.

Serves 8 to 10

*1 package dry yeast or 1 cake compressed yeast*
*¼ cup warm water*
*1 cup warm water or scalded milk, cooled to lukewarm*
*6 tablespoons honey or pure maple syrup*
*1 teaspoon salt*
*¼ cup uncolored butter or allowed margarine, softened*
*1 egg or equivalent egg replacer*
*1 cup wholewheat flour*
*3 to 3½ cups unbleached flour*
*½ cup uncolored butter or allowed margarine*
*6 tablespoons honey or pure maple syrup*
*1½ cups finely chopped nuts*

Preheat oven to 350°F

Dissolve yeast in ¼ cup warm water. Add 1 cup water or milk, sweetener, salt, shortening, and egg or egg replacer. Mix well. Stir in wholewheat flour and mix until smooth. Add enough of the unbleached flour so that the dough leaves the sides of the bowl. Knead on a floured board until the dough is very smooth. Put into a greased bowl. Turn the greased side up and cover. Let rise in a warm place until double in bulk, about 1½ hours. Punch down. Melt 3 tablespoons of shortening in bottom of an ungreased 10-inch tube pan. Add 2 tablespoons sweetener and mix. Melt the rest of shortening in a small pan. Stir in 2 tablespoons sweetener. Cut the dough into walnut-sized pieces with a scissors. Shape quickly into balls, and roll each in the shortening mixture in the small pan, then in the chopped nuts. Place the balls in tube pan, making two full layers in the pan. Drizzle the rest of the sweetener over the top. Cover and let rise until double in bulk, about 45 minutes. Bake for 30 to 35 minutes. As soon as cake is removed from the oven invert onto a plate and remove pan. Break cake into pieces with a fork when ready to serve.

### MUFFINS

(No milk, egg, corn, rye, or citrus)

Are you hungry for muffins but discouraged by the sugar used in muffin recipes? Just omit the sugar and top with allowed jam, honey butter, or pure maple syrup. Here's a typical muffin recipe, but the sugar is omitted and wheat germ is added to compensate for the white flour.

Makes 12 muffins

*1¾ cups unbleached flour*
*¼ cup toasted wheat germ*
*2½ teaspoons baking powder*
*1 teaspoon salt*
*⅓ cup melted uncolored butter or pure allowed vegetable oil*
*1 egg or equivalent egg replacer*
*1 cup milk or water*

Preheat oven to 400°F

Mix together dry ingredients. Combine remaining ingredients and add to dry ingredients. Stir just until dry ingredients are moistened. Fill greased muffin pans ⅔ full. Bake for 20 to 25 minutes.

**BLUEBERRY JAM OR SYRUP**

(No milk, egg, corn, wheat, rye, or citrus)

Here's some unsweetened blueberry jam to spread on those muffins or on toast, crackers, sandwiches, pancakes, or waffles. Instead of added sweeteners, this jam relies on the natural sweetness of the blueberries.

Makes 1 cup jam or 1¼ cups syrup

*1 pint fresh or frozen (thawed) blueberries*
*1½ cups water*

Mash blueberries in the bottom of a heavy saucepan. Add water. Cook over high heat until mixture boils. Reduce heat to low and simmer slowly to desired consistency. Use warm syrup on pancakes or waffles. Or refrigerate jam in a covered container

**GRAPE JAM**

(No milk, egg, corn, wheat, rye, or citrus)

This unsweetened grape jam will taste great on your peanut butter and jelly sandwiches. The pectin in the apple helps the jam to thicken.

Makes ½ cup

*4 cups purple grapes, washed*
*1 unwaxed apple, quartered and cored*
*½ cup water*
*2 cups bottled unsweetened grape juice*

Place grapes, apple, and water in a heavy saucepan. Bring to a boil. Reduce heat and simmer fruit until soft. Press soft fruit through a sieve, reserving juice and sieved pulp. Return juice and pulp to saucepan. Add bottled grape juice. Insert candy thermometer. Cook over medium heat until syrup reaches the sheeting stage (220° to 222°F) or when the jam on a spoon divides into two distinct drops that run together before falling from edge of spoon. Cool and refrigerate in a covered container.

### STRAWBERRY JAM

(No milk, egg, corn, wheat, rye, or citrus)

For fruits that aren't as sweet as blueberries and grapes, small amounts of honey, pure maple syrup, or fructose may be used to sweeten the jam.

Makes about 1¼ cups

*¼ cup honey or fructose*
*2 cups washed, quartered strawberries*
*1 unwaxed apple, peeled, cored, and sliced*
*¼ cup water*

Pour honey or fructose over prepared strawberries. Crush berries and let stand 15 minutes. In a large saucepan, combine sweetened strawberries, apple, and water. Bring to a boil over medium heat, stirring occasionally. Continue boiling until sheeting stage (220° to 222°F) is reached or when the jam on a spoon divides into two distinct drops that run together before falling from edge of spoon. Cool and refrigerate in a covered container.

### GELATIN SALAD OR DESSERT

(No milk, egg, corn, wheat, rye, or citrus)

You can still enjoy gelatin salads and desserts that are easy to make, attractive, delicious, nutritious, and free of all the junk found in commercial mixes. Tart juices such as lemon or grapefruit may be sweetened with a little honey or fructose.

Serves 4

*1 envelope unflavored gelatin*
*¼ cup cold water*
*1¾ cups unsweetened grape, pineapple, orange, or apple juice*
*1½ cups chopped fruits or vegetables*

In a small saucepan soften gelatin in cold water. Then warm over low heat until gelatin dissolves. Add to fruit juice and stir well. Chill. When almost set, stir in desired fruits or vegetables. Chill until firm. Do not use fresh pineapple as the gelatin won't set.

### SWEET PORK CHOPS

(No milk, egg, corn, wheat, rye, or citrus)

You can also use unsweetened fruit juices to add flavor and sweetness to meats and poultry. While you are satisfying your sweet cravings, you are also meeting your protein needs. Concentrated apple juice is used in this next recipe to make sweet, tasty pork chops.

Makes 4 1-inch thick pork chops

*4 pork chops, cut 1 inch thick*
*2 tablespoons pure allowed vegetable oil*
*¼ cup water*
*½ cup concentrated frozen apple juice, thawed*

Preheat oven to 350°F

In a heavy skillet, brown pork chops in oil. Place chops in an ovenproof dish. Add water. Season with salt and pepper. Spread concentrated apple juice on top of the chops. Cover and bake for 1 hour.

### APPLE OR PEAR PIE

(No milk, egg, corn, rye, or citrus)

Worried you'll have to give up apple pie? You can make delicious, sugar-free apple pie by selecting sweet apples and omitting any extra sweetener or by substituting honey or pure maple syrup. If by chance you're sensitive to apples, just substitute pears!

Makes 1 8- or 9-inch pie

*Double recipe Wheat Piecrust (see page 210)*
*6 cups peeled, sliced sweet apples or pears*
*½ teaspoon cinnamon*
*2 tablespoons unbleached flour*
*¼ to ½ cup honey or pure maple syrup (optional)*
*1 tablespoon uncolored butter or allowed margarine*

Preheat oven to 350°F

Arrange first piecrust in bottom of pie pan. Combine apples or pears with cinnamon and flour in bowl and toss lightly until thoroughly mixed. Place half of the fruit on the bottom crust and pour ⅛ to ¼ cup sweetener on top. Add the remaining fruit and drizzle sweetener over top. Dot with shortening. Cover with second crust, seal, and cut slits to let steam escape. Bake for 35 to 40 minutes until lightly browned and juices are bubbly. Cool before serving.

### WHIPPED TOPPING

(No egg, corn, wheat, rye, or citrus)

If your apple pie isn't complete without some whipped topping, this whipped cream is easy and delicious.

Makes about 2 cups

*½ teaspoon unflavored gelatin*
*1 tablespoon cold water*
*½ cup pure whipping cream*
*1 teaspoon pure vanilla extract*
*1 teaspoon honey or pure maple syrup (optional)*

In a small saucepan soften gelatin in cold water. Then warm over low heat until gelatin dissolves. Add to cream and stir well. Chill for 1 hour. Whip cream until it holds its shape. Add vanilla and sweetener. Refrigerate in a covered container until ready to use.

## VANILLA ICE CREAM

(No corn, wheat, rye, or citrus)
This vanilla ice cream uses honey as its sweetner.
Serves 6 to 8

*1 envelope unflavored gelatin*
*2 cups cold milk*
*⅓ cup honey*
*2 eggs, separated*
*⅛ teaspoon salt*
*2 teaspoons pure vanilla extract*
*2 cups half-and-half*

Sprinkle gelatin over cold milk in top of double boiler. Place over boiling water and stir until gelatin is dissolved. Add honey and stir until dissolved. Remove from heat. Add egg yolks and salt. Beat well with an electric mixer. Place again over boiling water and cook, stirring constantly until mixture coats spoon. Remove from heat. Cool. Stir in vanilla and cream. Pour into shallow pans and freeze until almost firm. Beat egg whites until stiff. Place frozen mixture in chilled bowl and beat until smooth. Fold in egg whites. Return to shallow pans and freeze until firm.

## ORANGE ICE CREAM

(No egg, corn, wheat, or rye)
Makes about 1 quart

*1 pint half-and-half*
*¾ cup pure unsweetened frozen (thawed) orange juice concentrate*
*2 tablespoons uncolored, unwaxed grated orange rind*

Combine cream and orange juice concentrate. Freeze in a tightly covered shallow pan until partially frozen. Scoop into a chilled bowl and beat until smooth but not melted. Fold in grated orange rind. Return to shallow pan. Cover tightly. Freeze until firm.

### PINEAPPLE ICE CREAM

(No egg, corn, wheat, rye, or citrus)

This ice cream recipe and the one for Orange Ice Cream (see page 221) use concentrated fruit juices and no other sweeteners. Use your ice cream maker if you have one, but you can easily make these recipes without one.

Makes about 1 quart

*1 pint half-and-half*
*3 ounces frozen (thawed) pineapple concentrate*
*1 cup chilled, well-drained unsweetened crushed pineapple*

Mix cream and pineapple concentrate together. Pour into a shallow pan. Cover tightly. Freeze until partially set. Scoop into a chilled bowl and beat until smooth but not melted. Fold in crushed pineapple and pour into a shallow pan. Cover tightly. Freeze until firm.

### MAPLE ICE CREAM

(No egg, corn, wheat, rye, or citrus)

Here's a yummy ice cream for special occasions made with pure maple syrup. Added peanut butter and dry milk powder make it more nutritious.

Makes 2 quarts

*2 cups pure whipping cream*
*1 cup milk*
*½ cup non-instant dry milk powder*
*¼ cup pure maple syrup*
*1 cup natural peanut butter*

In a large mixing bowl combine 1 cup whipping cream and milk. Beat in dry milk powder until well dissolved. Beat in maple syrup and peanut butter. In another bowl whip remaining cream until stiff. Fold into milk mixture. Freeze in a tightly covered shallow pan until partially frozen. Return to mixing bowl and beat until smooth but not melted. Return to freezer in the tightly covered shallow pan. Freeze until firm.

**STRAWBERRY ICE CREAM**

(No egg, corn, wheat, rye, or citrus)

This strawberry ice cream can be made with fructose or honey.

Makes almost 2 quarts

*1 quart (4 cups) strawberries*
*½ cup honey or fructose*
*1 cup milk*
*1½ teaspoons pure vanilla extract*
*2 cups pure whipping cream*

Wash strawberries well. Remove stems. Crush. Add sweetener and mix well. Add milk and vanilla. Mix well. Freeze in a tightly covered shallow pan until partially frozen. Whip cream. Beat strawberry mixture until smooth but not melted. Fold in whipped cream. Freeze until firm in a tightly covered shallow pan.

**YELLOW CAKE**

(No milk, egg, corn, rye, or citrus)

This plain yellow cake can be made with either honey or maple syrup.

Makes 1 9-inch round cake or 16 cupcakes

*1½ cups sifted unbleached flour*
*2 tablespoons wheat germ*
*2 teaspoons baking powder*

*½ teaspoon salt*
*¼ cup uncolored butter or allowed margarine, softened*
*⅓ cup honey or pure maple syrup*
*⅔ cup milk, water, or unsweetened pineapple juice*
*2 eggs or equivalent egg replacer*
*1½ teaspoons pure vanilla extract*

Preheat oven to 350°

Combine dry ingredients in one bowl. In another bowl cream together shortening and sweetener. Add liquid and egg or egg replacer. Beat in vanilla. Add flour mixture slowly. Beat for 2 minutes. Pour batter into a greased and lightly floured 9-inch round cake pan or into paper-lined cupcake pans, filling about ⅔ full. Bake cake for 20 minutes or until top springs back when lightly touched. Bake cupcakes for 15 minutes. Frost when completely cooled.

**CARROT CAKE**

(No milk, egg, corn, wheat, rye, or citrus)

You can even have your cake and eat it, too! Here's a carrot cake recipe that uses barley malt syrup, honey, or pure maple syrup for the sweetener. Carrots, pineapple, and raisins add extra sweetness.

Serves 10 to 12

*1 cup unbleached flour and 1 cup sifted wholewheat flour* or *¾ cup potato flour and ¾ cup rice flour*
*2 teaspoons baking powder*
*2 teaspoons baking soda*
*1 teaspoon cinnamon or allspice*
*1 cup pure allowed vegetable oil*
*¾ cup honey, pure maple syrup, or barley malt syrup*
*3 eggs or equivalent egg replacer*

*2 cups packed grated carrots*
*1 cup undrained, unsweetened, crushed canned pineapple*
*½ cup chopped walnuts*
*½ cup raisins*

Preheat oven to 350°F

In a large mixing bowl combine dry ingredients except nuts and raisins. Add oil, sweetener, and eggs or egg replacer, and beat until smooth. Stir in carrots, pineapple, walnuts, and raisins and mix thoroughly. Pour into a greased 9 × 13-inch cake pan and bake for 50 minutes. Wait 10 minutes before removing cake from pan. Cool and frost, if desired.

Frost these cakes with the Whipped Topping (see page 220). Or try one of these sugar-free icing recipes. The Fluffy Icing is like the kind you would make with corn syrup but uses honey instead.

### FLUFFY ICING

(No milk, corn, wheat, rye, or citrus)
Makes enough icing for 1 9-inch cake

*½ cup honey*
*2 egg whites*
*½ teaspoon pure vanilla extract*

In the top of a double boiler mix together honey and egg whites. Place over simmering water and beat with an electric mixer on medium-high speed for 10 to 12 minutes until stiff peaks form. Remove from heat and blend in vanilla.

**CREAM CHEESE FROSTING**
(No egg, corn, wheat, rye, or citrus)
Makes 1 cup

*1 8-ounce package cream cheese, softened*
*¼ cup honey or pure maple syrup*
*1 teaspoon pure vanilla extract*

Whip cream cheese. Slowly add sweetener. Beat in vanilla. Spread on cooled cake.

**FRUIT DROP COOKIES**
(No milk, egg, corn, rye, or citrus)
This nutritious cookie recipe can be made without any extra sweeteners because of the natural sweetness of the dates, apples, and fruit juice.
Makes about 40 cookies

*½ cup uncolored butter or allowed margarine, softened*
*½ cup date sugar or ¼ cup honey (optional)*
*2 eggs, slightly beaten, or equivalent egg replacer*
*1 cup chopped dates*
*1 coarsely grated apple or pear*
*1 cup rolled oats*
*½ cup chopped nuts*
*1½ cups unbleached flour*
*¼ cup toasted wheat germ*
*½ teaspoon cinnamon*
*½ teaspoon baking powder*
*¼ teaspoon salt*
*3 tablespoons unsweetened fruit juice (apple, pineapple, or pear)*

Preheat oven to 350°F

Cream shortening and sweetener. Add eggs or egg replacer and mix well. Stir in rest of ingredients. Drop by teaspoonfuls onto a greased cookie sheet. Bake for

12 minutes until lightly browned. Remove from cookie sheet immediately and cool thoroughly before storing.

**GINGER COOKIES**

(No milk, egg, corn, rye, or citrus)

Try adapting your favorite cookie recipes. Here are several examples. These ginger cookies are made with barley malt syrup or maple syrup instead of molasses.

Makes about 3 dozen cookies

*3/4 cup pure allowed vegetable oil, uncolored butter, or allowed margarine, softened*
*1/2 cup barley malt syrup or pure maple syrup*
*1 3/4 cups unbleached flour*
*1/4 cup toasted wheat germ*
*2 teaspoons baking soda*
*1/2 teaspoon salt*
*1/2 teaspoon cinnamon*
*2 teaspoons ginger*

Preheat oven to 350°F

In a large bowl cream together shortening and sweetener. In another bowl combine remaining ingredients. Mix together contents of both bowls and stir well. Drop by teaspoonfuls onto ungreased cookie sheet 3 inches apart. Flatten each with a fork or the palm of your hand. Bake for about 15 minutes. Remove from cookie sheet and let cool.

You'd give anything for an occasional piece of candy? Here are some suggestions using nuts, nut butters, and fruits for extra nutrition.

### CANDIED NUTS

(No milk, egg, corn, wheat, rye, or citrus)
Makes 2 cups

*½ cup pure maple syrup or honey*
*¼ cup water*
*1 tablespoon uncolored butter or allowed margarine*
*1¼ cups whole nuts*

Combine sweetener with water in a small heavy saucepan. Bring to a boil. Cook over medium heat until some syrup dropped into very cold water forms a firm ball when shaped with your fingers (242°). Remove syrup from heat and quickly stir in half the nuts. Drain nuts with slotted spoon and spread onto a greased plate. Repeat with remaining nuts. When cool, separate nuts.

### PEANUT BRITTLE

(No milk, egg, corn, wheat, rye, or citrus)
Makes about 90 1-inch pieces

*1⅓ cups pure maple syrup*
*⅔ cup water*
*¼ cup uncolored butter or allowed margarine*
*1 cup shelled peanuts*

In a medium saucepan combine maple syrup and water. Cook over medium heat until boiling. Add shortening and continue cooking, stirring frequently until some syrup dropped into very cold water forms a *soft* ball (234°). Add peanuts. Continue cooking, stirring frequently until some syrup dropped into very cold water now forms a *hard* ball (250°). Pour immediately onto a well-greased cookie sheet, spreading the candy around. When completely cool and candy is hard, loosen and crack into bite-sized pieces.

**PEANUT BUTTER FUDGE**
(No milk, egg, corn, wheat, rye, or citrus)
Makes about 1 pound

*1 cup pure maple syrup*
*2/3 cup milk, Soy Milk (see page 236), or Nut Milk (see page 236)*
*1/4 teaspoon salt*
*2 tablespoons uncolored butter or allowed margarine*
*1 teaspoon pure vanilla extract*
*1/2 cup smooth or crunchy natural peanut butter*
*3/4 cup chopped walnuts, pecans, or peanuts*

Combine maple syrup, milk, salt, and shortening in a heavy saucepan. Bring to a boil over medium heat. Continue cooking and stirring until some syrup dropped into very cold water forms a soft ball (234°). Remove from heat. Add vanilla and peanut butter and beat with an electric mixer until fudge begins to stiffen. Fold in nuts. Turn into lightly greased loaf pan. Cool. Cut into pieces.

**FRUIT SNACKS**
(No milk, egg, corn, wheat, rye, or citrus)
Makes 25 pieces

*1 cup chopped dried apricots*
*1 cup raisins or currants*
*1/2 cup finely chopped nuts*
*1/2 cup toasted wheat germ or ground nuts*
*1 cup shredded unsweetened coconut*
*1/4 cup honey*

Mix all ingredients together. Form into balls, adding more honey if necessary to make the balls keep their shape. Store in covered container.

**FRUIT LEATHER**
(No milk, egg, corn, wheat, rye, or citrus)
Makes 6 large pieces

*5 or 6 large pieces of ripe, sweet-tasting fruit (apples, peaches, pears, plums, bananas, apricots, or nectarines)*

Preheat oven to 170°F

Wash fruit thoroughly. Cut out any blemishes. Cut into chunks and put into a blender on high speed until smooth. Lightly grease an 11 × 17-inch jelly roll pan. Pour fruit onto the pan and spread evenly. Put into the oven but leave the door slightly ajar to let moisture escape. Leave in the oven until the fruit has dried evenly all over and can be lifted from the pan. Cut into pieces. Store in an airtight container.

**STUFFED DATES**
(No milk, egg, corn, wheat, rye, or citrus)
Makes 12 pieces

*12 dates*
*12 walnut halves*
*¼ cup cream cheese, softened (optional)*

Slit dates lengthwise. Insert part of a walnut or a whole nut if dates are large. Or fill date with cream cheese. Refrigerate in covered container.

**FRUIT JUICE POP**
(No milk, egg, corn, wheat, rye, or citrus)
Soda pop that's nutritious? Try this.
Makes 8 ounces

*4 ounces unsweetened grape juice, pure unsweetened orange juice, or pineapple juice*
*4 ounces soda water or Perrier water*

Combine juice and soda water. Serve over ice cubes.

Is your Fourth of July incomplete without lemonade? Here are two recipes to try.

### APPLE LEMONADE

(No milk, egg, corn, wheat, or rye)
Makes about 2 cups

*2 cups pure unsweetened apple juice*
*4 tablespoons pure lemon juice*

Combine juices. Chill. Serve over ice.

### LEMONADE

(No milk, egg, corn, wheat, or rye)
Makes 7 8-ounce servings

*8 ounces pure lemon juice*
*½ cup honey*
*6 cups cold water*
*1 uncolored unwaxed lemon, sliced (optional)*

In a blender combine lemon juice and honey on high speed. Mix with cold water in a large pitcher. Add lemon slices, if desired. Serve over ice.

You don't have to give up canning or freezing your favorite fruits just because you can't use sugar. Here are some general directions.

### CANNING FRUITS

1) Prepare fruit. Pack firmly into sterilized glass jar.
2) Pour water into jar to level suggested by jar manufacturer. Or use ½ teaspoon sodium ascorbate crystals (a form of vitamin C) dissolved in 1 quart of boiling water to prevent fruit from discoloring. Or use thinned apple juice or white grape juice. Or prepare more juice made from the fruit you're canning.

3) Slide sterilized knife along edge of jar to remove air bubbles.
4) Screw tops and lids on firmly.
5) Process in water-bath or under pressure as designated by general canning instructions.

**FREEZING FRUITS**

1) Add ½ teaspoon sodium ascorbate crystals to 1 quart of water. Cover sliced fruit with the liquid, pressing fruit down with a small piece of crumbled parchment paper to hold it under the liquid. Or pack crushed or sliced fruit in its own juice without any sweetener. Or use other unsweetened fruit juices like orange, apple, white grape, pineapple, or papaya.
2) Cover, seal, and freeze.

**STRAWBERRY SOFT-SERVE**

(No egg, corn, wheat, rye, or citrus)

A new low-calorie sweetener, aspartame, sold under the trade name Equal may also be helpful in preparing foods that don't have to be baked or heated at high temperatures since aspartame is destroyed by heat. Ice cream, puddings, jams, gelatin molds, and cold beverages all can be made well with Equal. For example, you can use Equal to make this tasty soft-serve ice cream.

Serves 4

*1 package frozen unsweetened strawberries (do not thaw)*
*½ pint whipping cream or half-and-half*
*4 packages Equal*

Place all ingredients in blender. Blend until smooth. Serve immediately.

## ASPARTAME STRAWBERRY JAM

(No egg, corn, wheat, rye, or citrus)

Use Equal to sweeten homemade jams, but remember you can't cook it at high heats. So don't add the Equal until the jam has cooled. Gelatin is used to thicken the jam.

Makes 2 cups

*½ package (1½ teaspoons) unflavored gelatin*
*2 tablespoons cold water*
*1 20-ounce package frozen unsweetened strawberries (thawed), plus juice*
*6 to 8 packets Equal*

Soften gelatin in cold water. Bring strawberries and juice to a boil. Reduce heat and simmer until soft. Add softened gelatin and stir until completely dissolved. Cool. Stir in Equal. Refrigerate.

## PUMPKIN PIE

(No corn, wheat, rye, or citrus)

You can even make aspartame-sweetened pies by cooking the crust separately, cooking the filling on top of the stove, letting it cool, then stirring in the Equal, and pouring the filling into the crust. You can even make two-crust pies by cooking a top crust (a circle of dough slightly less than the diameter of the pie is cooked on a cookie sheet) separately, then adding it last to the rest of the finished pie. Try this single crust pumpkin pie sweetened with Equal.

Makes 1 8- or 9-inch pie

*1 recipe allowed piecrust, baked and cooled*
*1½ cups cooked pumpkin*
*1½ cups half-and-half*
*½ teaspoon salt*
*1 teaspoon cinnamon*

*½ teaspoon ginger*
*½ teaspoon nutmeg*
*3 slightly beaten eggs*
*1 envelope unflavored gelatin*
*¼ cup water*
*8 packages Equal*

In the top of a double boiler mix together pumpkin, cream, salt, spices, and eggs. Cook over, not in, hot water until filling thickens. In the meantime, soften gelatin in cold water. Then warm over low heat until gelatin dissolves. Add to pumpkin mixture and stir well. Refrigerate pumpkin filling until it begins to thicken. Stir in Equal. Pour into prepared piecrust. Cover and refrigerate until filling is set.

### CAROB MILK

(No egg, corn, wheat, rye or citrus)

Or you can use Equal to sweeten beverages such as this carob milk drink.

Makes 8 ounces

*8 ounces cold milk*
*1 tablespoon carob powder*
*1 to 2 packets Equal*
*⅛ teaspoon pure vanilla extract*

Mix together all the ingredients.

# 16

# Cooking Without Milk

## MILK SUBSTITUTES

If tolerated, substitute goats' milk for cows' milk in appropriate recipes. However, you may not like the strong taste of the goats' milk.

If tolerated, substitute for 1 cup milk, ½ cup commercial soy milk and ½ cup water in appropriate recipes.

For evaporated milk, substitute commercial soy milk cup for cup.

If you find the taste of soy milk objectionable, try adding 1 teaspoon lime juice per cup to take away the strong nutty flavor.

Substitute Banana, Nut, Oat or Soy Milk for milk cup for cup in appropriate recipes.

In baking, for 1 cup milk substitute 1 cup water or 1 cup allowed fruit juice plus 1 tablespoon extra oil or shortening.

For 1 cup sour cream, mix 4 tablespoons allowed starch with ¾ cup water. Then stir in ¼ cup vinegar. Use in casseroles.

For milk, substitute chicken stock cup for cup in cream soups and casseroles.

There are lots of different substitutions for milk, but you'll soon get the knack of which one will taste best in a given recipe. Here are several recipes for milk substitutions you can make at home. Nut or banana milk is good on cereals, but banana milk must be used immediately before it darkens.

**BANANA, NUT, OR OAT MILK**
(No milk, egg, corn, wheat, rye, or citrus)
Makes 1 cup

*½ small banana or ⅓ cup nuts or seeds (cashews, walnuts, sliced almonds, sunflower seeds, sesame seeds) or 2 teaspoons rolled oats.*
*1 cup water.*

Combine banana, nuts, seeds, or oats and water in blender on highest speed until smooth.

**SOY MILK**
(No milk, egg, corn, wheat, rye, or citrus)
Makes 7 cups

*½ pound (1¼ cups) dry soybeans*
*8 cups water*

Soak beans in 4 cups water for at least 12 hours. Drain well and discard water. Place half the beans in a blender. Add 2 cups water. On high speed finely grind the beans. Repeat with other half of the beans and another 2 cups water. Heat mixture in a heavy saucepan over medium heat, stirring frequently until temperature reaches 131°F or is too hot to touch comfortably. Cool. Strain mixture through a cloth, reserving all the liquid. Heat this liquid in the top of a double boiler for 45 minutes, stirring frequently. Add enough water to make, in all, 7 cups soy milk. Keep refrigerated.

### MILK-FREE WHIPPED TOPPING

(No milk, egg, corn, wheat, rye, or citrus)

Gelatin makes this milk-free substitute for whipped cream creamy and fluffy.

Makes 4 cups

*2 envelopes unflavored gelatin*
*½ cup cold water*
*1 cup honey*
*¾ cup boiling water*
*½ teaspoon salt*
*1 teaspoon pure vanilla extract*
*¼ cup ice water*

Soften gelatin in cold water. In a 2-quart heavy saucepan add honey to boiling water. Continue boiling until syrup reaches the thread stage (230° to 234° F, when syrup forms thread as it is dropped from the edge of a spoon). Remove from heat.

Add softened gelatin to hot syrup and stir until dissolved. Cool 10 to 15 minutes. Add salt and vanilla. Beat with mixer until mixture becomes thick and cool. Add ice water and continue beating until fluffy.

Store sauce in a covered container in the refrigerator. If sauce is too thick, it may be thinned by heating in the top of double boiler over hot water and beating until fluffy and creamy.

### MILK-FREE PANCAKES

(No milk, egg, corn, wheat, rye, or citrus)

Instead of using milk in waffles, pancakes, or biscuits, substitute water or unsweetened pineapple juice.

Makes 10 pancakes

*1¼ cups wholewheat flour or rye flour*
*3 teaspoons baking powder*
*½ teaspoon salt*

*1 egg, beaten, or 2 tablespoons water and ½ teaspoon baking powder*
*1 cup plus 2 tablespoons milk, unsweetened pineapple juice, or water*
*2 tablespoons pure allowed vegetable oil*

Stir together dry ingredients. Stir together liquid ingredients and add to dry ingredients. Stir until just mixed. Bake on greased griddle or in a lightly oiled skillet. Batter may be thinned as needed with extra milk, water, or juice. Serve hot with syrup or allowed homemade jam.

**TOMATO SOUP**
(No milk, egg, corn, wheat, rye, or citrus)
For delicious, creamy soups, substitute chicken stock for milk.
Makes 1 pint

*1 6-ounce can tomato paste*
*2 cups Chicken Stock (see page 209)*
*¼ teaspoon instant minced onion*
*¼ teaspoon celery salt*
*¼ teaspoon salt*
*1 tablespoon honey*

In a large saucepan combine all ingredients. Bring to a boil and then simmer for 5 minutes.

**FISH CHOWDER**
(No milk, egg, corn, wheat, rye, or citrus)
Makes 2 quarts

*1 cup finely diced carrots*
*1 cup diced uncooked potatoes*
*1 cup chopped onion*
*½ cup finely diced celery*
*1 bay leaf*

*1 12-ounce package frozen (thawed) fish fillets*
*1/4 cup pure allowed vegetable oil*
*1/4 cup unbleached flour or rice flour*
*2 teaspoons salt*
*3 1/2 cups Chicken Stock (see page 209)*
*Dried parsley flakes*

In a large saucepan place carrots, potatoes, onion, celery, and bay leaf. Add water to cover and bring to a boil. Turn to simmer and cook 15 minutes. Add fish and cook 15 minutes longer. With a fork break fish into small chunks. Discard bay leaf. Cover pan and set aside.

Heat oil in another saucepan, add flour and salt, and mix. Stir in stock or milk gradually. Cook over medium heat, stirring constantly until mixture bubbles. Combine with fish mixture. Serve hot with sprinkling of parsley flakes.

**CREAMED CHICKEN**

(No milk, egg, corn, wheat, rye, or citrus)

Instead of a milk-based white sauce, this creamed chicken uses chicken stock.

Serves 4

*2 tablespoons pure allowed vegetable oil*
*2 tablespoons unbleached flour or rice flour*
*1 cup Chicken Stock (see page 209)*
*1/2 teaspoon salt*
*1/8 teaspoon paprika*
*1 teaspoon frozen or dried chives*
*2 cups diced cooked chicken*

In a saucepan, mix oil and flour. Add stock and bring to a boil, stirring constantly. Add salt, paprika, and chives. Stir in chicken and simmer for a few minutes until chicken is heated. Stir so the sauce does not stick to the pan. Serve mixture over rice, noodles, or atop buttered toast.

### MASHED POTATOES

(No milk, egg, corn, wheat, rye, or citrus)

Baking powder makes these mashed potatoes light and fluffy.

Makes 4 servings

*4 medium white potatoes*
*1 tablespoon uncolored butter or allowed margarine*
*4 teaspoons baking powder*
*Salt and pepper to taste*

Scrape white potatoes. Cook until soft in boiling salted water. Drain thoroughly. Add allowed shortening and seasoning. Mash. Add baking powder (1 teaspoon per potato) and continue mashing until fluffy. Season to taste.

### COCONUT PUDDING

(No milk, corn, wheat, rye, or citrus)

This pudding uses coconut milk to make a tasty dessert.

Serves 4

*2 cups shredded unsweetened coconut*
*3 cups boiling water*
*1 tablespoon unflavored gelatin*
*3 egg yolks*
*3 tablespoons honey*

Put coconut into a heat-proof bowl. Pour the boiling water over the coconut and allow to sit until lukewarm. Drain coconut through a fine sieve or cheesecloth, reserving all liquid. Squeeze the coconut until thoroughly drained. Liquid should measure 2 cups. If necessary, add water to make the 2 cups.

Pour coconut liquid into a saucepan and mix with the other ingredients. Cook over medium heat until very hot and gelatin is dissolved. Do not boil. Pour into serving dishes and refrigerate 3 to 4 hours until set. Divide ½ cup of the drained coconut into 4 equal portions and stir into each partially set portion of pudding.

**MAPLE APPLE OR PEAR PUDDING**

(No milk, egg, corn, wheat, rye, or citrus)

This pudding substitutes water for milk and uses tapioca as its thickener.

Serves 6

*3 tablespoons quick-cooking tapioca*
*⅛ teaspoon salt*
*2 tablespoons pure maple syrup*
*⅓ cup cold water*
*½ cup chopped dates*
*¼ cup chopped nuts*
*½ cup raisins*
*1½ cups sliced apples or pears, peeled if waxed*
*1½ cups boiling water*

In the top of a double boiler, combine tapioca, salt, maple syrup, and cold water. Let stand 5 minutes. Add remaining ingredients and mix well. Cook over boiling water until pudding is thickened and fruit is tender. Serve plain or with allowed topping.

**SOY PUMPKIN ICE CREAM**

(No milk, egg, corn, wheat, rye, or citrus)

Are you screaming for ice cream? This maple ice cream is made from commercial soy milk. The pumpkin and spices disguise the soy flavor while adding extra nutrition. Carefully read the label on the soy milk to make sure it doesn't contain any corn, cow's milk, or sugar.

Makes about 1 quart

*1 13-ounce can concentrated soy milk*
*¾ cup water*
*1 cup pumpkin*
*¼ teaspoon salt*
*⅔ cup maple syrup*
*¼ teaspoon nutmeg*
*¼ teaspoon cinnamon*

With electric mixer or blender, thoroughly blend all ingredients. Pour into shallow pans. Cover tightly. Freeze until partially frozen. Scoop into a bowl and beat until light. Return to pans. Cover tightly. Freeze until firm.

**FRUIT ICE**

(No milk, egg, corn, wheat, rye, or citrus)

Try this fruit ice as a cool refreshing substitute for ice cream

Serves 4

*1 envelope unflavored gelatin*
*¼ cup cold water*
*2 cups unsweetened grape juice, orange juice, or pineapple juice*
*2 tablespoons honey (optional)*

Soften gelatin in cold water in a small saucepan. Then stir over low heat until gelatin dissolves. Add to fruit juice and mix well. Stir in honey. Pour into a 9-inch square pan and freeze until frozen around the edges. In a chilled bowl, beat the partially frozen fruit ice until smooth but not melted. Return to pan. Cover tightly with foil. Freeze until firm.

### TOFU CHEESE SPREAD

(No milk, egg, corn, wheat, rye, or citrus)

Looking for a nutritious cheesy snack? Try this "cheese" spread made from tofu (soybean curd), available in the produce department of many grocery stores.

Makes ¼ cup

*4 tablespoons tofu*
*4 tablespoons chopped chives*
*1 teaspoon salt*

Blend ingredients thoroughly. Serve on crackers or spread on celery stalks.

### MILK-FREE EGGNOG

(No milk, corn, wheat, rye, or citrus)

Finally, for a nutritious milk-free eggnog, this recipe substitutes fruit juice for milk.

Serves 2

*2 cups unsweetened orange juice or pineapple juice*
*1 to 2 eggs*
*2 teaspoons pure lemon juice (optional)*

Combine ingredients and mix well in a blender or with an electric mixer. Serve over cracked ice.

# 17

# Cooking Without Eggs

## EGG SUBSTITUTES

Omit eggs in appropriate recipes. Cookies and quick breads often turn out well without any eggs.

Use commercial egg replacer such as Jolly Joan Egg Replacer. Follow directions on box. Be sure to check list of ingredients on egg replacers to ensure the product is egg-free.

Use Soy Egg Yolk Substitute (see page 246) as directed.

Use Apricot Egg Replacer (see page 245) as directed.

Use 1 tablespoon cornstarch to replace 1 egg in making custard.

Substitute for 1 egg: 2 tablespoons allowed starch, ½ tablespoon allowed shortening, ½ teaspoon baking powder plus 2 tablespoons liquid.

When making egg-free cookies, grease and lightly flour the cookie sheet to prevent cookies from spreading.

When baking an egg-free cake, the flavor and texture changes can be disguised by adding or increasing ingredients such as raisins, nuts, or spices.

If a recipe is egg-free, milk-free, and wheat-free, the baking time should be longer on a lower heat.

Cooking without eggs is difficult in some types of recipes. Eggs act as leavening agents, making the finished product lighter. Eggs also bind ingredients together, keeping the finished product from crumbling. If you also have to substitute for some other common ingredients like milk, sugar, and flour, you often end up with a heavy product or one that falls apart. The above tips and the following illustrative recipes should help you cook without eggs.

**APRICOT EGG REPLACER**

(No milk, egg, corn, wheat, rye, or citrus)

This can be used in cookies, muffins, meat loaf, and quick breads to help bind the ingredients together.

Makes 1¼ cups

*6 ounces sun-dried apricots*
*1½ cups water*

Cook apricots in water until soft. Cool. Puree in the blender. Keep refrigerated in a covered container. Use 2 tablespoons apricot egg replacer for each egg. Add extra ½ teaspoon baking powder per egg to make batters rise in appropriate recipes.

### SOY EGG YOLK SUBSTITUTE

(No milk, egg, corn, wheat, rye, or citrus)
This can be used for binding purposes.
Makes 1½ cups

*1 cup soy powder or soy flour*
*2 cups water*
*2 tablespoons pure allowed vegetable oil*
*¼ teaspoon salt*

Thoroughly blend powder and water in a blender on high speed. Pour into the top of a double boiler and cook over boiling water, covered, for about 1 hour. Beat in oil and salt with an electric mixer. Refrigerate. Will thicken when cooled. Use about ¼ cup of the soy substitute for each egg. An extra ½ teaspoon baking powder per egg can be added to make batter lighter.

### EGG-FREE MAYONNAISE

(No milk, egg, corn, wheat, rye, or citrus)
Mayonnaise is made with eggs to emulsify the oil. But you can make an egg-free mayonnaise with the following recipe
Makes 1 cup

*1½ tablespoons rice flour or 2 tablespoons unbleached flour*
*½ teaspoon salt*
*¼ teaspoon dry mustard*
*¼ cup cold water*
*¾ cup boiling water*
*1 tablespoon allowed vinegar*
*½ cup pure allowed vegetable oil*
*⅛ teaspoon paprika*
*Salt and pepper*

Combine flour, salt, dry mustard, and cold water in a saucepan. Stir until smooth. Add boiling water. Stir constantly over medium heat until mixture thickens and comes to a boil.

Cool until lukewarm. Combine vinegar and oil. Add the vinegar and oil very slowly to the mixture, beating constantly. When it is well blended, beat in paprika. Add salt and pepper to taste. Refrigerate in a covered container.

Egg-free mayonnaise is used as you would regular mayonnaise. For instance, use it in this vegetable dip.

### VEGETABLE DIP

(No milk, egg, corn, wheat, rye, or citrus)
Makes 1 cup

*1 cup Mayonnaise (see page 202) or Egg-Free Mayonnaise (see page 246)*
*1 teaspoon curry powder*
*¼ teaspoon dry mustard*
*½ teaspoon garlic salt*
*½ teaspoon onion salt*
*2 drops Tabasco sauce*

Combine all ingredients and chill. Serve as a dip with raw vegetables.

### POTATO SALAD

(No milk, egg, corn, wheat, rye, or citrus)
This potato salad can be made with regular mayonnaise or egg-free mayonnaise. The hard-cooked eggs can be omitted.
Serves 5 to 6

*1 cup Mayonnaise (see page 202) or Egg-Free Mayonnaise (see page 246)*
*1 teaspoon dry mustard*
*2 teaspoons pure lemon juice (optional)*

*¼ teaspoon celery seed*
*½ teaspoon onion salt*
*5 cups cubed cold cooked potatoes*
*3 hard-cooked eggs, chopped (optional)*
*½ cup chopped celery*
*Salt and peper to taste*

Combine first five ingredients and mix well. Place potatoes, chopped eggs, and celery in a large bowl and pour mayonnaise mixture on top. Toss lightly until dressing is evenly distributed. Adjust seasonings by adding salt and pepper to taste.

---

**PEANUT BUTTER COOKIES**

(No milk, egg, corn, rye, or citrus)

These peanut butter cookies hold together well without any eggs or egg replacer.

Makes 3½ dozen cookies

*½ cup pure maple syrup or honey*
*½ cup pure allowed vegetable oil or uncolored butter or allowed margarine, softened*
*1 teaspoon pure vanilla extract*
*1 cup natural peanut butter*
*1½ cups unbleached flour*
*¼ cup toasted wheat germ*
*¼ teaspoon salt*
*½ teaspoon baking soda*
*½ teaspoon baking powder*

Preheat oven to 375°F

In a large bowl combine maple syrup, shortening, and vanilla. Beat until well mixed. Add peanut butter and mix well. In a small bowl combine flour, wheat germ, salt, baking soda, and baking powder. Add dry ingredients to wet and mix well. Drop dough from teaspoon onto ungreased cookie sheet and press flat with a fork. Bake for about 15 minutes. Remove from cookie sheet and let cool completely.

**REFRIGERATOR COOKIES**

(No milk, egg, corn, rye, or citrus)

These refrigerator cookies are also made without eggs to bind them together.

Makes 4 dozen cookies

*1 cup pure allowed vegetable oil, uncolored butter, or allowed margarine, softened*
*¾ cup pure maple syrup or honey*
*2 teaspoons pure vanilla extract*
*½ cup toasted wheat germ*
*2 cups unbleached flour*
*1 cup wholewheat flour*
*2 teaspoons baking powder*
*1 teaspoon salt*
*1 teaspoon baking soda*
*1 cup chopped nuts (optional)*

Preheat oven to 400°F

In a large bowl, cream together shortening and sweetener. Stir in vanilla. In another bowl, combine dry ingredients except nuts. Add dry ingredients to shortening mixture, combine, and then add nuts. Wrap dough in waxed paper and chill 4 hours or overnight. When ready to bake, shape dough into walnut-sized balls and place on greased cookie sheet. Flatten each ball with a fork. If the edges crumble, press them together. Cookies may be decorated with nuts, dried fruits, raisins, or seeds. Bake for 8 to 10 minutes; remove from cookie sheet while still warm.

**CARROT RAISIN COOKIES**

(No milk, egg, corn, wheat, rye, or citrus)

These carrot raisin cookies substitute extra baking powder and water for the eggs. To keep these cookies from spreading too much (especially when using oat flour) lightly four the greased cookie sheet.

Makes 5 dozen cookies

*1 cup wholewheat flour or oat flour*
*2 cups rolled oats*
*½ cup wheat germ (optional)*
*1½ teaspoons baking powder*
*1 teaspoon salt*
*¾ cup honey*
*½ cup uncolored butter or allowed margarine, softened*
*2 eggs or an extra teaspoon baking powder plus ¼ cup water*
*1½ cups packed finely grated carrots*
*1 cup raisins*
*½ cup chopped walnuts or pecans*

Preheat oven to 350°F

Combine all ingredients in a large bowl. Mix well. Drop by teaspoonfuls onto a greased and lightly floured cookie sheet and bake 12 minutes or until lightly browned. Remove from cookie sheet immediately and let cool. Store in an airtight container.

**CHEESECAKE**

(No egg, corn, wheat, rye, or citrus)

Many cheesecake recipes call for eggs. Instead, this recipe uses gelatin to make the cake set.

Serves 8

*1 recipe any allowed piecrust*
*1 cup boiling water*
*1 envelope unflavored gelatin*
*¼ cup honey*

*2 8-ounce packages cream cheese, softened*
*1 teaspoon pure vanilla extract*
*1 cup sour cream (optional)*
*Fresh fruit (optional)*

Prepare a piecrust for a 9-inch pie pan (including baking if needed). Cool if just baked. In a large bowl pour boiling water over gelatin and stir until completely dissolved. Add honey and stir well. With an electric mixer beat in cream cheese and vanilla until smooth. Pour cheese mixture into crust. Chill in refrigerator until firm. Top, if desired, with sour cream or sliced fresh fruit.

**GINGERBREAD**

(No milk, egg, corn, wheat, rye, or citrus)

The spices in this gingerbread help disguise the different texture and flavor that result when cooking without eggs and wheat.

Makes 1 8-inch square cake

*⅔ cup honey*
*½ cup melted uncolored butter or allowed margarine*
*¾ teaspoon cinnamon or allspice*
*¾ teaspoon nutmeg*
*1 teaspoon ginger*
*½ cup boiling water*
*2½ cups unbleached flour or 3 cups oat flour*
*1 teaspoon baking soda*

Preheat oven to 350°F

Combine honey, shortening, and spices. Stir in boiling water. Mix in flour. Add baking soda and stir until thoroughly mixed. Pour into a well-greased and lightly floured 8-inch square pan. Bake 30 to 35 minutes or until a toothpick inserted in the center comes out clean. Let cool 4 minutes in pan. Turn out on wire rack.

## EGG-FREE CAROB CAKE

(No milk, egg, corn, wheat, rye, or citrus)

This easy carob cake gets its leavening power from baking soda and vinegar. Cooling it in the pan for 10 minutes is important so that it doesn't break apart when you remove it.

1 8-inch square cake

*1½ cups sifted unbleached flour, or 2 cups Scotch-style oatmeal or oat flour*
*1 teaspoon baking soda*
*½ teaspoon salt*
*2 tablespoons carob powder*
*1 teaspoon pure vanilla extract*
*1 tablespoon allowed vinegar*
*5 tablespoons uncolored butter or allowed margarine, melted*
*½ cup honey*
*1 cup water*

Preheat oven to 350°F

Combine all dry ingredients. Add vanilla, vinegar, and melted shortening. Mix well. Stir in honey and water and mix well until all ingredients are well blended. Batter will be thin. Pour into a lightly greased and floured 8-inch square cake pan. Bake 40 to 45 minutes or until a toothpick inserted in the center comes out clean. Cool in pan 10 minutes. Carefully remove and cool thoroughly on wire rack.

# 18

# Cooking Without Corn, Wheat, or Rye

## CORN, WHEAT, AND RYE SUBSTITUTES

Corn Substitutes:

1 cup corn syrup = ½ cup pure maple syrup or ½ cup honey

For thickening, 1 tablespoon cornstarch =

- 1 tablespoon arrowroot
- 2 tablespoons wheat flour
- 1 tablespoon potato starch flour
- 1 tablespoon rice flour
- 4 teaspoons quick-cooking tapioca

Wheat and Rye Substitutes (⅝ cup = ½ cup plus 2 tablespoons):

In baking, 1 cup wheat flour =

- 1 cup rye flour
- ½ cup arrowroot
- ½ cup barley flour

¾ cup buckwheat
1 cup corn flour
1⅓ cups ground oats or oat flour
⅝ cup potato starch or potato flour
¾ to ⅞ cup rice flour
1⅓ cups soy flour
1 cup tapioca flour
⅝ cup rice flour + ⅓ cup potato flour
½ cup rye flour + ½ cup potato flour
⅝ cup rice flour + ⅓ cup rye flour
1 cup soy flour + ¼ cup potato starch
½ cup cornstarch + ½ cup rye flour
½ cup cornstarch + ½ cup potato flour

For thickening, 1 tablespoon wheat flour =
1½ teaspoons arrowroot
1½ teaspoons potato starch
1½ teaspoons rice flour
2 teaspoons quick-cooking tapioca

Spaghetti and Noodle Substitutes:
Chinese bean threads
Rice
Rice flour noodles
Spaghetti squash
Rice Vermicelli

While a corn-free diet is difficult because corn products are so prevalent in prepared foods, corn-free cooking is easy. Simply omit whole corn from appropriate recipes like soups and stews. Use maple syrup or honey instead of corn syrup. Substitute another starch for cornstarch when a thickening agent is needed. Commercial baking powder usually contains cornstarch so if you can't find a corn-free one, you can make the baking powder in Chapter 14.

### TOASTED RICE

(No milk, egg, corn, wheat, rye, or citrus)

Do you miss snacking on popcorn? Bag this toasted rice and take it to the next movie.

Makes 4 cups

*4 cups puffed rice cereal or crumbled rice cakes*
*½ cup uncolored butter or allowed margarine, melted*
*Salt*

Preheat oven to 350°F

Spread rice in a shallow baking pan. Sprinkle lightly with shortening. Salt to taste. Toast until lightly brown, about 10 minutes.

### CARAMEL RICE

(No milk, egg, corn, wheat, rye, or citrus)

For a sweeter treat, try this substitute for caramel corn.

Makes about 2 quarts

*½ cup uncolored butter or allowed margarine, melted*
*½ cup honey or pure maple syrup*
*2 quarts puffed rice cereal or crumbled rice cakes*
*½ cup chopped nuts or seeds*

Preheat oven to 350°F

Blend shortening and sweetener in a saucepan. Heat over medium heat until mixture begins to bubble. Pour over rice and nuts in a large bowl. Toss quickly to coat rice and nuts evenly. Spread on 2 ungreased cookie sheets. Bake about 10 to 15 minutes until crisp and lightly browned.

### VANILLA PUDDING

(No egg, corn, wheat, rye, or citrus)

Homemade puddings call for cornstarch to make them thicken. Try potato starch instead. Potato starch requires less simmering than flour or cornstarch and should not be allowed to boil as the pudding will thin out. Potato starch doesn't hold as well as cornstarch or flour, so puddings should be eaten as soon as possible. Potato starch may also be used to thicken soups and gravies.

Serves 6

*¼ cup cornstarch or potato starch flour*
*¼ teaspoon salt*
*2¼ cups milk*
*¼ cup honey or pure maple syrup*
*2 tablespoons uncolored butter or allowed margarine*
*1 teaspoon pure vanilla extract*

In a large saucepan combine cornstarch or potato starch and salt. Add milk slowly and stir until smooth. Stir in sweetener. Cook over medium heat stirring constantly. For potato starch pudding, remove from heat as soon as pudding thickens. For cornstarch pudding, bring to a boil and continue boiling and stirring for 1 minute. Stir in shortening and vanilla and mix well. Refrigerate in a covered container.

### PINEAPPLE PUDDING

(No milk, egg, corn, wheat, rye, or citrus)

This pineapple pudding uses arrowroot as the thickener. Arrowroot powder is tasteless and thickens at a lower temperature than wheat flour or cornstarch. It is also ideal for cream sauces and clear, delicate glazes.

Serves 4

*1 20-ounce can unsweetened chunk or crushed pineapple, drained, reserving juice*
*1½ tablespoons arrowroot*
*1 banana, sliced (optional)*

Measure 1 cup drained pineapple and set aside. Liquefy rest of pineapple and juice in blender. Pour into a heavy saucepan. Add arrowroot powder and mix well. Cook over medium heat, stirring constantly until pudding thickens. Remove from heat. Stir in crushed or chunk pineapple and banana slices. Chill.

**BLUEBERRY PIE**

(No milk, egg, corn, rye, or citrus)

Quick-cooking tapioca can also be used to thicken gravies, sauces, fruit fillings, clear glazes, and puddings. Overcooking will cause stringiness. Don't boil. Sauces will thicken after removal from heat. This blueberry pie is thickened with tapioca.

Makes 1 8- or 9-inch pie

*Double recipe Wheat Piecrust (see page 210)*
*4 cups fresh, canned, or frozen (thawed) blueberries*
*1 tablespoon water*
*1 tablespoon pure lemon juice (optional)*
*¼ cup honey*
*3½ tablespoons quick-cooking tapioca or 4½ tablespoons unbleached flour*
*2 tablespoons uncolored butter or allowed margarine*

Preheat oven to 375°F

Prepare piecrust, but do not prebake. Combine blueberries, water, lemon juice, and honey in a heavy saucepan. If using tapioca, add tapioca and let stand 10 minutes. Cook over medium heat until berries are tender. If not using tapioca, add flour. Stir until filling thickens over medium heat. Cool. Pour into prepared pie shell. Dot with shortening. Cover with top crust and seal edges. Slit top crust with knife in several places. Bake for about 30 minutes or until crust is golden brown.

A wheat-free diet is difficult because wheat is the basis for so many different foods—breads, crackers, cereals, spaghetti, pies, cakes, cookies, and so on. But there are lots of other flours and starches you can substitute for wheat.

**ALL-RYE BREAD**

(No milk, egg, corn, wheat, or citrus)

Baking yeast bread without wheat is difficult because other grains have little or no gluten, which is what gives wheat its elastic quality. So don't expect soft, light loaves. If you tolerate rye, RyKrisp crackers can be used for a tasty crunchy sandwich. This all-rye bread is good for toast or sandwiches.

Makes 2 loaves

*3 packages dry yeast* or *3 cakes compressed yeast*
*2½ cups warm water or milk*
*2 teaspoons salt*
*4 tablespoons pure allowed vegetable oil*
*1 tablespoon honey (optional)*
*1 tablespoon caraway seeds*
*4½ to 5 cups rye flour*
*Uncolored butter or allowed margarine*

Preheat oven to 350°F

Dissolve yeast in warm liquid. Stir in salt, oil, honey, and caraway seeds. Add 2 cups flour and stir well. Cover and let rise for ½ hour. Add 2 cups flour a little at a time. Dough will be stiff. Cover and let rise 1½ hours. Sprinkle ½ cup flour over a flat surface. Knead flour into dough a little at a time until dough is no longer sticky. Add more rye flour, if necessary. Knead about 5 to 8 minutes. Divide dough in two and shape into loaves. Place on greased baking sheet. Brush loaves with shortening. Cover and let rise, about 2 hours. Bake for 1 hour or until loaf sounds hollow when tapped on the bottom.

### FRIED BREAD

(No milk, egg, corn, wheat, rye, or citrus)

This fried bread has a yeasty taste but gets its leavening power from the baking powder. Oat flour is easily made by finely grinding rolled oats in a blender.

Makes 28 rolls

*1 package dried yeast* or *1 cake compressed yeast*
*2 cups warm water*
*2 to 4 tablespoons honey*
*2 cups whole wheat flour and 2 cups unbleached flour* or *5 to 5⅓ cups oat flour*
*1 teaspoon salt*
*5 teaspoons baking powder*
*Pure allowed vegetable oil*

Sprinkle yeast over water. Stir in honey. Mix together all dry ingredients. Add yeast and honey mixture to dry ingredients. Mix well. Pat dough out on a floured surface until it is about ¾ inch thick. Use additional flour to avoid stickiness. Tear or cut off pieces about the size of a small biscuit. Deep fry in allowed oil at 365°F. Turn to brown on both sides. Be certain that bread is done in the center and not doughy. Serve hot with allowed butter or margarine and/or desired jam or fruit butters.

### SWEET RYE OR OAT BREAD

(No milk, egg, corn, wheat, or rye)

This sweet-tasting bread makes delicious toast. The flavor improves with age, but the bread may be eaten right away.

Makes 1 loaf

*2 cups rye flour or oat flour*
*½ teaspoon baking soda*
*2 teaspoons baking powder*
*½ teaspoon salt*
*1 tablespoon cinnamon* or *1 extra teaspoon allspice*
*½ teaspoon allspice*
*¼ teaspoon nutmeg*
*½ cup honey or pure maple syrup*
*¾ cup plus 2 tablespoons water*
*1 tablespoon pure unsweetened frozen (thawed) orange juice concentrate*
*1 tablespoon grated uncolored unwaxed orange rind*
*½ cup finely chopped nuts (optional)*

Preheat oven to 350°F

Combine dry ingredients except nuts. Mix together sweetener and water in a saucepan and heat until mixture just starts to boil. Pour over dry ingredients. Beat with an electric mixer for 5 minutes. Beat in orange juice, orange rind, and nuts. Batter will be thick. Spread evenly in a greased 8½ × 4½-inch loaf pan. Place a pan of water on lowest oven rack. Place loaf pan on rack above. Bake for 1 hour. Remove from pan and cool on wire rack. Wrap well in foil to store.

### PUMPKIN BREAD

(No milk, egg, corn, wheat, rye, or citrus)

Wheat-free batter breads work well because the other

ingredients disguise the taste and texture of the substituted flours.

Makes 1 loaf

*1⅛ cups rice flour* or *2 cups unbleached flour*
*½ cup honey*
*½ teaspoon cinnamon*
*½ teaspoon salt*
*¼ teaspoon nutmeg*
*1 teaspoon baking soda*
*½ teaspoon baking powder*
*¾ cup canned pumpkin*
*¼ cup pure allowed vegetable oil*
*½ cup water*
*½ cup chopped nuts*
*¼ cup wheat germ (optional)*

Preheat oven to 350°F

Combine all ingredients in a large mixing bowl. Mix until just blended. Pour batter into greased 9 × 5 × 3-inch loaf pan. Bake 50 to 60 minutes or until a toothpick inserted in the center comes out clean. Cool in pan for 10 minutes. Turn out onto wire rack. Cool completely.

**ZUCCHINI BREAD**

(No milk, egg, corn, wheat, rye, or citrus)

Makes 1 loaf

*1⅛ cups rice flour or 1¼ cups unbleached flour and ¼ cup wheat germ*
*½ teaspoon baking soda*
*½ teaspoon salt*
*¼ teaspoon nutmeg*
*½ teaspoon cinnamon*
*3 tablespoons water*
*1 egg (optional)*

*⅓ cup pure allowed vegetable oil*
*1 teaspoon pure vanilla extract*
*½ cup honey*
*1 cup chopped zucchini, peeled if waxed*
*¼ cup chopped nuts*

Preheat oven to 350°F

In a large bowl mix together flour, baking soda, salt, nutmeg, and cinnamon. Add water, egg, oil, vanilla, and honey. Beat until thoroughly blended. Stir in zucchini and nuts. Pour into a 9 × 5 × 3-inch greased loaf pan. Bake for 50 to 55 minutes. Let cool in the pan. Remove from pan and cool completely.

**RICE STUFFING**

(No milk, egg, corn, wheat, rye, or citrus)

Instead of stuffing chicken or turkey with bread stuffing, use rice as the base.

Makes enough stuffing for two 3½-pound chickens

*2 tablespoons uncolored butter or allowed margarine*
*½ cup minced onion*
*2 4-ounce cans mushroom pieces, drained*
*2 to 3 cups cooked brown rice*
*½ teaspoon poultry seasoning*

Melt shortening in a heavy skillet and sauté onion until partially cooked. Add mushroom pieces and cook for several more minutes. Add rice and poultry seasoning. Mix thoroughly. Stuff chickens and cook as directed. Any leftover stuffing can be heated in the oven in a covered dish.

**CORN MUFFINS**

(No milk, wheat, rye, or citrus)

If you tolerate corn, these corn muffins are wheat-free.

Adding the cornmeal to boiling water avoids graininess.

Makes 12 medium-sized muffins

*1 cup stone-ground cornmeal*
*1½ cups water*
*2 tablespoons uncolored butter or allowed margarine, melted*
*¾ teaspoon salt*
*1 egg*
*2 teaspoons baking powder*

Preheat oven to 425°F

Add cornmeal to 1 cup boiling water. Remove from heat. Stir in shortening, salt, egg, baking powder, and ½ cup water. Spoon into 12 medium-sized greased muffin pans. Bake for 15 to 20 minutes.

### WHEAT-FREE MUFFINS

(No milk, corn, wheat, or citrus)

These muffins use a combination of oats and rye flour. A combination of flours will improve both taste and texture of wheat-free products.

Makes 16 muffins

*2 cups rolled oats*
*1 cup rye flour*
*2 teaspoons baking powder*
*2 teaspoons baking soda*
*½ teaspoon salt*
*¾ cup unsweetened apple juice*
*¼ cup honey*
*¼ cup pure allowed vegetable oil*
*2 eggs*
*¾ cup chopped fruit (currants, diced apples, pears, raisins, dates, drained unsweetened crushed canned pineapple, dried apricots, etc.) (optional)*

Preheat oven to 350°F

Combine dry ingredients. Add all other ingredients and stir until thoroughly mixed. Fill greased muffin cups half full and bake 15 minutes until lightly browned.

### RICE MUFFINS

(No milk, egg, corn, wheat, rye, or citrus)

These muffins use rice flour instead of corn or wheat.

Makes 9 muffins

*1½ cups rice flour*
*2 teaspoons baking powder*
*½ teaspoon baking soda*
*½ teaspoon salt*
*⅔ cup milk or water*
*2 tablespoons honey*
*1 tablespoon pure allowed vegetable oil*
*1 egg or equivalent egg replacer*
*¾ cup fresh or frozen (thawed) blueberries (optional)*

Preheat oven to 350°F

Combine all ingredients except blueberries in a mixing bowl. Stir until thoroughly blended. Gently fold in blueberries. Fill greased muffin tins one-half full. Bake until lightly browned, about 20 minutes. Remove from pan while still hot. Serve warm.

### POTATO PANCAKES

(No milk, egg, corn, wheat, rye, or citrus)

These potato pancakes can be served for breakfast or dinner.

Makes 8 pancakes

*4 medium potatoes, coarsely grated*
*4 tablespoons unbleached flour or rice flour*

*2 teaspoons salt*
*1 egg or 4 tablespoons Mayonnaise (see page 202) or Egg-Free Mayonnaise (see page 246)*

Combine all ingredients until thoroughly blended. Fry on a greased griddle until lightly browned on both sides.

### OAT OR RICE PANCAKES

(No milk, egg, corn, wheat, rye, or citrus)

If breakfast seems incomplete without pancakes, don't despair. Pancakes can be made from a variety of different flours. Because of their size, it's not as difficult to get wheat-free pancakes to stick together as it is wheat-free breads and cakes. Some allergic persons who live on rotation diets have found they can have pancakes every morning by rotating the flour, liquids, oils, and toppings they use! Try these oat or rice pancakes.

Makes 6 medium pancakes

*1 cup oat flour or rice flour*
*1 teaspoon baking powder*
*½ teaspoon baking soda*
*1 teaspoon salt*
*1 egg or equivalent egg replacer*
*2 tablespoons pure allowed vegetable oil*
*½ cup milk, Soy Milk (see page 236), unsweetened apple juice, or water*

Combine all ingredients and mix until smooth. Add more liquid if necessary until you get a fairly thin batter. Cook on a lightly greased griddle until browned on both sides. Serve hot with honey, jam, or maple syrup.

**GRANOLA CEREAL OR BARS**

(No milk, egg, corn, wheat, rye, or citrus)

If you enjoy cereal for breakfast but you can't have wheat, try oatmeal, cream of rice, cream of rye, or puffed rice. Or make this wheat-free granola.

Makes 10 cups

*4 cups rolled oats*
*1 cup toasted sesame seeds*
*1 cup toasted wheat germ (optional)*
*1 cup shredded unsweetened coconut*
*1 cup chopped nuts*
*2 cups raisins or currants*
*½ cup pure maple syrup*
*½ cup honey*
*¼ cup pure allowed vegetable oil*

Preheat oven to 250°F

Combine all dry ingredients (including nuts and raisins) in a large bowl. Mix the sweeteners and oil together and pour over dry ingredients while stirring. Continue to stir until well mixed. Spread granola out on two or three lightly greased cookie sheets and bake in the oven for 30 minutes, stirring about every 10 minutes. Allow the cereal to cool on the baking sheets and then store in airtight containers.

To make the mixture into bars, press into the bottom of baking pans until about ⅜ inch deep. Bake in the oven for 30 minutes. As soon as you remove the granola from the oven cut into bars of desired size with a sharp knife. Allow to cool in the pans. Remove and store bars in airtight containers.

## COTTAGE CHEESE CRACKERS

(No egg, corn, wheat, rye, or citrus)

Just about all commercial crackers contain wheat. These crackers are made with rice flour.

Makes about 2 dozen crackers

*1⅛ cups rice flour or 1½ cups unbleached four*
*¾ teaspoon salt*
*½ cup uncolored butter or allowed margarine, softened*
*½ cup additive-free cottage cheese*

Preheat oven to 450°F

In a large bowl mix flour and salt. Add softened shortening and cottage cheese. Cut in with pastry blender until well blended. Wrap dough in waxed paper and refrigerate for at least 1 hour.

On a well-floured board, roll out dough to ⅛-inch thickness. Cut out crackers with a 2-inch cookie cutter and place on ungreased baking sheet. Prick each cracker with a fork. Bake for 12 to 15 minutes until lightly browned. Remove from baking sheet and cool on a rack.

## OAT CRACKERS

(No milk, egg, corn, wheat, rye, or citrus)

Oat flour is the base for these crackers.

Makes 1 to 1½ dozen crackers

*1 cup oat flour*
*½ teaspoon salt*
*¼ teaspoon baking soda*
*4 tablespoons cold water*
*2 tablespoons pure allowed vegetable oil*
*1 tablespoon cold water (if needed)*

Preheat oven to 375°F

In a small bowl combine flour, salt, and baking soda. Add water and oil and mix well. Add an additional tablespoon of cold water if needed to make a soft dough. Shape into a ball. Roll dough as thin as possible on a board sprinkled with oat flour. Cut with a cookie cutter or cut into rectangles with a sharp knife. Place on a lightly greased cookie sheet. Bake for 3 minutes, turn once and bake 3 minutes longer or until lightly brown and crisp.

**RICE CAKE SNACKS**

(No milk, egg, corn, wheat, rye, or citrus)

You should be able to locate rice cakes at your grocery or health foods store. They're not really cakes but are more like a cracker made from puffed rice. If you don't like them plain, try these suggestions.

*Rice cakes*
*Uncolored butter or allowed margarine*
*Onion salt, celery salt, or grated Parmesan cheese*

Preheat oven to 350°F

Spread each cake with uncolored butter or allowed margarine. Sprinkle with one of the following: onion salt, celery salt, or grated Parmesan cheese. Place on a cookie sheet. Heat for 2 to 3 minutes.

Or the rice cakes may be spread with peanut butter and lightly toasted under the broiler. Serve warm.

**WHEAT-FREE SPAGHETTI**

(No milk, egg, corn, wheat, rye, or citrus)

What can be done to satisfy wheat-sensitive spaghetti and pizza lovers? First, try serving allowed spaghetti sauce over rice. Or try spaghetti sauce over spaghetti squash.

Serves 3 to 4

*1 3½- to 4-pound spaghetti squash*
*2 cups allowed spaghetti sauce*
*Parmesan cheese (optional)*

Preheat oven to 350°F

Cut squash lengthwise and scoop out seeds. Place halves face down in a shallow dish and add about ½ inch water. Bake in oven for 45 minutes to 1 hour or until soft when pricked with a fork. Remove from oven. Drain thoroughly. Scoop squash from shell by running the tines of a fork lengthwise down the squash pulp so that it comes out in spaghetti-like strings. Top with sauce and Parmesan cheese, if allowed.

### WHEAT-FREE PIZZA

(No egg, corn, wheat, rye or citrus)

For wheat-free pizza try this: top a toasted rice cake with a slice of mozzarella cheese. Melt cheese under the broiler. Top cheese with a thin layer of allowed pizza sauce, meat, and another cheese slice. Melt cheese under the broiler and serve immediately. Or try this recipe where mashed potatoes substitute for the usual wheat crust.

Makes 1 9-inch pizza

*1 tablespoon uncolored butter or allowed margarine*
*3 cups cold mashed potatoes (4 medium potatoes)*
*⅔ cup allowed spaghetti or pizza sauce*
*½ pound ground beef or pork, browned*
*4 ounces mozzarella cheese, shredded*

Preheat oven to 400°F

Grease a 9-inch pie pan with allowed shortening. Press mashed potatoes into the bottom and up the sides. Bake for about 15 to 20 minutes until lightly browned. Top with sauce, meat, then cheese. Return pizza to oven for another 5 to 10 minutes until cheese is melted and bubbly.

### FRIED CHICKEN

(No milk, egg, corn, wheat, rye, or citrus)

Wheat flour or crumbs are the basis for all coating and breading mixes. Oat or rice flour is substituted for wheat flour in this recipe for fried chicken.

Serves 4 to 6

*1 cup unbleached flour, wholewheat flour, oat flour, or rice flour*
*2 teaspoons salt*
*1 teaspoon poultry seasoning*
*1 2½- to 3-pound frying chicken, cut up*
*1 cup milk or water*
*½ cup pure allowed vegetable oil*
*¼ cup water*

In a plastic bag combine the flour, salt, and poultry seasoning. Dip chicken in milk or water and shake a few pieces at a time in bag with flour until well coated. Heat oil in skillet and brown chicken on all sides. Reduce heat, add water, cover, and continue to cook chicken about 40 to 45 minutes or until tender. Remove cover and cook an additional 10 minutes until crispy.

Chicken can be cooked after browning by placing pieces on cookie sheet and baking in the oven for 45 minutes at 350°F. This gives a very crisp crust.

### COCONUT CRUST

(No milk, egg, corn, wheat, rye, or citrus)

Here are some suggestions for wheat-free piecrusts. It's difficult to make a wheat-free double crust that you can roll out for both a top and bottom crust. Non-wheat flours just don't stick together very well.

Instead, if you need a top crust, double the recipe, fit half into the bottom of the pie pan and crumble the other half on top.

Makes 1 8- or 9-inch crust

*3 tablespoons uncolored butter or allowed margarine*
*1½ cups shredded unsweetened coconut*
*1 tablespoon honey*

Preheat oven to 350°F

Grease pie pan with 1 tablespoon shortening. Melt remaining shortening and combine thoroughly with coconut and honey, using your fingers if necessary. Pour into pie pan and press mixture around the sides and bottom until evenly distributed. Bake in oven 8 to 10 minutes until lightly browned. Cool and fill.

### NUT CRUST

(No milk, egg, corn, wheat, rye, or citrus)
Makes 1 8- or 9-inch piecrust

*1⅓ cups finely chopped nuts (walnuts or pecans)*
*2 tablespoons butter or allowed margarine, melted*

Preheat oven to 350°F

Mix together the nuts and shortening. Press against the sides and bottom of pie pan, using the back of a spoon. Bake for 12 minutes. Cool before filling.

### RICE PIECRUST

(No milk, egg, corn, wheat, rye, or citrus)
Makes 1 8-inch crust

*¾ cup rice flour*
*½ teaspoon salt*
*3 tablespoons pure allowed vegetable oil*
*¼ cup cold water*

Preheat oven to 350°F

In a small bowl combine flour and salt. Add oil and water. Mix thoroughly and shape into a ball. Place in the middle of an 8-inch pie pan. Gently flatten the dough and press it up the sides of the pan. Bake for 15 to 20 minutes. Cool before filling.

### RYE CRUMB CRUST

(No milk, egg, corn, wheat, or citrus)

Makes 1 8-inch or 9-inch piecrust

*1½ cups RyKrisp or Wasa cracker crumbs*
*½ cup uncolored butter or allowed margarine, melted*
*3 tablespoons pure maple syrup or honey*
*1 teaspoon cinnamon*

Preheat oven to 350°F

Mix cracker crumbs with shortening, sweetener, and cinnamon. Pat firmly into pie pan. Bake for 5 to 7 minutes. Cool before filling.

### APPLE OR PEAR CRISP

(No milk, egg, corn, wheat, rye, or citrus)

This apple crisp dessert is easily prepared with any allowed fruit and may be served warm or cold.

Serves 4

*5 to 6 apples or pears*
*½ cup oat flour*
*¼ cup uncolored butter or allowed margarine*
*2 tablespoons pure maple syrup*

Preheat oven to 375°F

Peel, core, and slice fruit. Place in a deep dish. Mix together other ingredients working quickly so the mixture does not become oily. Spread on top of fruit. Bake for 45 minutes or until fruit is done and the topping is lightly browned.

### OATMEAL CAKE

(No milk, corn, wheat, rye, or citrus)

Non-wheat flours work best in cakes if you can use eggs to help them stick together. A combination of flours is more palatable than one flour. A lower baking temperature and a long baking time are usually better. Wheat-free cakes tend to be dry. Frosting, fruits, and nuts help to keep cakes moist and improve their taste and texture.

This oatmeal cake uses both rolled oats and oat flour for a better texture.

Makes 1 13 × 9-inch cake

*1 cup rolled oats*
*½ cup uncolored butter or allowed margarine*
*¾ cup honey*
*1¼ cups boiling water*
*1 teaspoon pure vanilla extract*
*2 eggs*
*1¾ cups unbleached flour or oat flour*
*1 teaspoon baking soda*
*¾ teaspoon salt*
*1 teaspoon cinnamon and ¼ teaspoon nutmeg* or ½ teaspoon extra pure vanilla extract

Preheat oven to 350°F

Place oats, shortening, honey, and boiling water in a large bowl. Stir. Let stand 20 minutes. Beat in vanilla and eggs. Mix together remaining ingredients and beat them into batter. Pour into a greased and floured 13 × 9-inch pan. Bake 30 to 40 minutes or until a toothpick inserted in the center comes out clean. May be iced but is good plain.

**APPLESAUCE CAKE**

(No milk, egg, corn, wheat, rye, or citrus)

This spicy cake can be made with potato starch flour. Nuts and applesauce improve the texture.

Makes 1 9-inch round cake

*½ cup uncolored butter or allowed margarine*
*⅓ cup honey or pure maple syrup*
*1 egg, slightly beaten, or ½ teaspoon baking powder and 2 tablespoons water or unsweetened juice*
*1½ cups unsweetened applesauce*
*2 cups unsifted unbleached flour or 1½ cups potato starch flour*
*1½ teaspoons cinnamon or allspice*
*½ teaspoon nutmeg*
*½ teaspoon salt*
*1 teaspoon baking soda*
*1 teaspoon pure vanilla extract*
*1 cup nuts (optional)*

Preheat oven to 350°F

Cream together shortening and sweetener. Add egg or egg substitute and applesauce. Mix well. Stir in dry ingredients except nuts. Beat well, using an electric mixer for several minutes. Beat in vanilla. Stir in nuts. Pour into a greased and floured 9-inch round cake pan. Bake about 40 minutes or until a toothpick inserted in the center comes out clean and cake starts to pull away from sides of pan. Cool in pan on wire rack for 5 minutes. Turn out on rack. Serve plain or frost with desired icing.

**FRUIT CAKE**

(No milk, corn, wheat, rye, or citrus)

Fruits, nuts, and eggs keep this cake moist and disguise the nonwheat flour.

Makes 2 5 × 9-inch cakes

*1½ cups raisins*
*1½ cups currants*
*1½ cups chopped dates*
*1½ cups chopped dried apricots*
*1½ cups chopped walnuts*
*2 8-ounce cans unsweetened crushed canned pineapple, including juice*
*1 cup uncolored butter or allowed margarine*
*½ cup pure maple syrup*
*6 eggs*
*3 cups wholewheat flour, rye four, or 2¼ cups rice flour*
*1 teaspoon baking powder*
*1 tablespoon cinnamon*
*1 teaspoon nutmeg*
*½ teaspoon allspice*
*½ cup water*

Preheat oven to 300°F

Combine first six ingredients, mix thoroughly and let stand 1 hour. Cream together shortening and maple syrup. Add eggs and beat well. Combine dry ingredients and add to shortening mixture alternately with water. Stir in nut and fruit mixture and mix well. Pour into greased 5 × 9-inch loaf pans. Bake for 1½ hours. Remove from pans and cool completely. Store in airtight containers.

Cookies are easier to make than cakes without wheat flour. Their size helps to keep them from crumbling. The same tips suggested for cakes apply to cookies. Here are some sample recipes. Now adapt your favorite recipes!

**PUMPKIN COOKIES**

(No milk, egg, corn, wheat, rye, or citrus)

Makes 3½ dozen cookies

*1½ cups wholewheat flour or rye flour*
*½ teaspoon baking powder*
*½ teaspoon baking soda*
*¼ teaspoon cinnamon*
*¼ teaspoon nutmeg*
*1 teaspoon salt*
*½ cup uncolored butter or allowed margarine, softened*
*⅓ cup pure maple syrup*
*1 egg or equivalent egg replacer*
*½ cup pure unsweetened apple juice*
*1 teaspoon pure vanilla extract*
*1 cup canned pumpkin*
*1 cup chopped nuts*

Preheat oven to 350°F

Blend together all dry ingredients except nuts and set aside. Cream together shortening and maple syrup. Add egg or egg replacer, apple juice, vanilla, and pumpkin. Stir in dry ingredients and then chopped nuts. Drop by teaspoonfuls onto ungreased cookie sheet and bake 15 minutes. Remove from cookie sheet and let cool completely.

**OATMEAL COOKIES**

(No milk, egg, corn, wheat, rye, or citrus)

Makes about 40 cookies

*¾ cup uncolored butter or allowed margarine, softened*
*½ cup honey*
*1 egg (optional)*
*¼ cup milk or water*

*1 teaspoon pure vanilla extract or 1 teaspoon pure orange extract and 1 teaspoon uncolored unwaxed orange rind*
*1 cup unbleached flour or oat flour*
*1 teaspoon salt*
*½ teaspoon baking soda*
*3 cups rolled oats*
*½ cup raisins, chopped nuts, or unsweetened flaked coconut (optional)*

Preheat oven to 350°F

Cream together shortening and honey. Beat in egg and liquid. Add vanilla extract or orange extract and rind. Mix in flour, salt, and baking soda. Work in oats. Add raisins, nuts, or coconut. Drop from teaspoon onto a greased (and floured if making recipe without egg) cookie sheet. Bake for about 12 minutes or until cookies are lightly browned. Let cookies cool on cookie sheet for 1 minute. Remove. Let cookies cool completely.

### LEMON DATE MACAROONS

(No milk, corn, wheat, or rye)
Makes 5 dozen cookies

*1 cup uncolored butter or allowed margarine, softened*
*¾ cup honey*
*2 eggs*
*¼ cup pure lemon juice*
*¾ cup chopped dates*
*½ cup chopped nuts*
*1 cup sifted unbleached flour, rice flour, or oat flour*
*½ teaspoon salt*
*1 teaspoon baking soda*
*3 cups rolled oats*

Preheat oven to 350°F

Cream shortening and honey together. Mix in eggs and lemon juice. Beat thoroughly. Stir in dates and nuts. Add flour, salt, and soda. Mix well. Add oats and mix thoroughly. Measure level tablespoons of dough and put on a well-greased cookie sheet. Press mounds flat. Bake for 12 to 15 minutes. Remove from cookie sheet and let cool.

# 19

# Cooking Without Chocolate

## CHOCOLATE SUBSTITUTES

Replace cocoa with carob powder measure for measure.

Replace 1 square of unsweetened chocolate with 3 tablespoons carob powder plus 1 to 1½ extra tablespoons pure allowed vegetable oil, allowed margarine, or uncolored butter.

Replace chocolate chips with finely chopped dried fruits such as apricots, figs, and especially dates in appropriate recipes.

Chocolate lovers who are allergic to chocolate take heart! Carob is a healthy, delicious, easy, naturally sweet substitute for chocolate. It's easy to substitute carob for chocolate by using the guide above. The following recipes will help you adapt your own chocolaty treats.

## CAROB ICE CREAM

(No corn, wheat, rye, or citrus)

If you can't live without your chocolate ice cream, try this carob ice cream as an occasional treat.

Serves 6 to 8

*Vanilla Ice Cream (see page 221)*
*6 to 8 tablespoons carob powder*

Prepare ice cream as directed but dissolve carob powder in hot milk containing the dissolved gelatin.

## CAROB SYRUP

(No milk, egg, corn, wheat, rye, or citrus)

This carob syrup can be used in milk shakes, for making "chocolate" milk, sodas, or as a sauce on ice cream.

Makes 1½ cups

*6 tablespoons pure maple syrup or honey*
*½ cup carob powder*
*¼ teaspoon salt*
*1 cup milk or Soy Milk (see page 236)*
*2 teaspoons pure vanilla extract*

Combine sweetener, carob powder, salt, and milk in a heavy saucepan. Stir until smooth. Bring to a boil over medium heat, stirring constantly. Reduce heat and continue cooking and stirring for 1 minute.

Remove pan from heat. Add vanilla. Cool to room temperature, then refrigerate.

## CAROB FUDGE SAUCE

(No milk, egg, corn, wheat, rye, or citrus)

For a thick carob "fudge" sauce, try this.

Makes 1¼ cups

*¾ cup carob powder*
*¼ teaspoon salt*
*⅔ cup milk or Soy Milk (see page 236)*
*½ cup honey*
*2 tablespoons uncolored butter or allowed margarine*
*1 teaspoon pure vanilla extract*

Combine carob powder and salt in a medium saucepan. Slowly stir in milk and honey and mix until smooth. Add shortening. Bring to a boil over medium heat, stirring constantly. Cook over low heat, stirring frequently, for 5 to 7 minutes, until very thick. Remove from heat and stir in vanilla. Let cook and store in covered container in refrigerator. Serve cold or reheat in a double boiler.

### CAROB PUDDING

(No egg, corn, wheat, rye, or citrus)

If creamy chocolate pudding is a favorite, this carob pudding should ease your chocolate cravings.

Serves 6

*Vanilla Pudding (see page 256)*
*2 to 4 tablespoons carob powder*

Prepare vanilla pudding as directed. Add carob powder when vanilla is added. Stir until well mixed and carob is melted. Refrigerate in a covered container.

### CAROB COOKIES

(No milk, egg, corn, rye, or citrus)

This nutritious carob cookie will take your mind off your dreams of chocolate chip cookies.

Makes about 3 dozen cookies

*½ cup uncolored butter or allowed margarine, softened*
*⅓ cup honey*
*¼ cup water*
*2 tablespoons toasted wheat germ*
*1 cup unbleached flour*
*¼ cup carob powder*
*1 teaspoon baking powder*
*¼ teaspoon baking soda*
*¼ teaspoon salt*
*1½ teaspoons pure vanilla extract*
*½ cup chopped walnuts or pecans*
*½ cup chopped dates*

Preheat oven to 400°F

Cream together shortening and honey. Mix in water. Combine dry ingredients except nuts and dates and add to creamed mixture. Mix well. Add vanilla, nuts, and dates. Stir well. Drop by teaspoonfuls onto a greased cooked sheet. Bake 8 to 10 minutes. Remove from cookie sheet and let cool.

### CAROB CAKE

(No milk, corn, rye, or citrus)

Turn your favorite chocolate cake recipe into a carob cake substituting carob for cocoa and honey or pure maple syrup for the sugar.

Makes 2 9-inch-round layers

*½ cup uncolored butter or allowed margarine, softened*
*¾ cup honey*
*2 eggs*
*⅓ cup carob powder*
*⅓ cup water*
*2 cups sifted unbleached flour*
*1 teaspoon baking powder*

*1 teaspoon baking soda*
*½ teaspoon salt*
*⅔ cup buttermilk, milk, or water*
*1½ teaspoons pure vanilla extract*
*⅔ cup chopped nuts or dates (optional)*

Preheat oven to 350°F

Cream well together shortening and honey. Add eggs, beating until fluffy. Blend carob powder with water. Stir into shortening and egg mixture. In another bowl combine dry ingredients except nuts or dates. Add to creamed mixture alternately with the buttermilk or other liquid, beating well. Add vanilla and nuts or dates. Mix thoroughly. Bake in two greased and floured 9-inch layer cake pans for 25 to 35 minutes. Cool in pans on wire racks for 10 minutes. Turn out on racks. Cool completely. Ice with desired frosting.

## CAROB FROSTING

(No egg, corn, wheat, rye, or citrus)
Frost your cake with this fluffy carob icing.
Makes about 1½ cups

*1 teaspoon unflavored gelatin*
*½ pint pure whipping cream*
*2 tablespoons carob powder, sifted*
*½ teaspoon pure vanilla extract*
*3 packages Equal*

In a small saucepan soften gelatin in ¼ cup cream. Then warm over low heat until gelatin dissolves. Add to balance of cream. Stir in carob powder, vanilla, and Equal. Mix thoroughly. Chill. Beat with an electric mixer on high speed until icing is fluffy and holds its shape well. Spread on cooled cake. Keep refrigerated until serving time. Refrigerate leftovers.

**HOT CAROB DRINK**

(No egg, corn, wheat, rye, or citrus)

Do you miss your hot chocolate on a cold, snowy evening? This hot carob drink may be just what you need.

Serves 2

*2 cups milk*
*3 tablespoons carob powder*
*2 teaspoons honey (optional)*

Combine all ingredients in a saucepan and stir until well mixed. Heat and continue stirring until carob powder is dissolved and mixture is desired temperature.

**CAROB BROWNIES**

(No milk, corn, rye, or citrus)

Do you have a favorite brownie recipe? Try substituting carob powder for the cocoa or unsweetened chocolate and honey or pure maple syrup for the sugar.

Makes 16 brownies

*¾ cup unbleached flour*
*¼ cup toasted wheat germ*
*1 teaspoon baking powder*
*¼ teaspoon salt*
*½ cup carob powder, sifted*
*½ cup uncolored butter or allowed margarine, melted*
*⅔ cup honey*
*2 eggs, well beaten*
*1 teaspoon pure vanilla extract*
*½ cup chopped nuts*

Preheat oven to 350°F

Combine flour, wheat germ, baking powder, and salt and mix well. In a large bowl, add carob powder to melted butter; stir in honey, then blend in beaten eggs. Add flour mixture and blend thoroughly. Stir in vanilla and nuts and mix well. Spread in a greased 8-inch square pan. Bake 25 minutes. Brownies are done when a toothpick inserted in the center comes out clean. Cool. Cut into 16 squares.

**CAROB FUDGE**

(No milk, egg, corn, wheat, rye, or citrus)

If you just have to have something sweet and chocolaty, try this carob fudge. Nuts, wheat germ, and dry milk powder make it more nutritious than most fudge.

Makes 24 ounces or 64 pieces

*½ cup carob powder*
*¾ cup milk or water*
*¾ cup honey*
*¼ cup uncolored butter or allowed margarine*
*1 teaspoon pure vanilla extract*
*1 cup chopped nuts*
*¼ cup toasted wheat germ*
*1½ to 1¾ cups non-instant dry milk powder or potato starch flour*

In a heavy saucepan combine carob, liquid, honey, and shortening. Bring to a rolling boil over medium heat and continue boiling for 2 minutes. Remove from heat and cool. Stir in vanilla, nuts, and wheat germ. Work in milk powder or potato starch until candy is thick. Press into a greased 8-inch square pan. Cover and refrigerate until firm. Cut into pieces. Keep refrigerated.

# 20

# Cooking Without Tomatoes

Good news! Just because you're allergic to tomatoes, you don't have to give up your catsup, spaghetti, or lasagna! Here are some ways to avoid tomatoes.

First, here is a chili recipe that's tasty without tomatoes.

**TOMATOLESS CHILI**
(No milk, egg, corn, wheat, rye, or citrus)
Serves 4 to 6

*½ pound dried kidney beans*
*1 large onion, chopped*
*1 green pepper, chopped*
*1 pound ground beef*
*1½ tablespoons chili powder*
*1½ teaspoons salt*
*¼ teaspoon pepper*
*1 bay leaf*
*⅛ teaspoon paprika*
*½ cup water*
*¼ cup unbleached flour or rice flour*
*Parmesan cheese for topping (optional)*

Prepare dried kidney beans according to directions on package. In a large skillet brown onion, green pepper, and beef. Add cooked beans, including the liquid in which they were cooked. Add chili powder, salt, pepper, bay leaf, and paprika. Simmer, covered, 1½ hours. Just before serving, make a paste of water and flour and add to chili if it is too thin. Good with grated Parmesan cheese sprinkled on top.

**BAKED BEANS**

(No milk, egg, corn, wheat, rye, or citrus)

This baked bean recipe also avoids using tomato sauce or catsup.

*1 cup dry navy beans*
*3½ cups water*
*¼ teaspoon parsley flakes*
*1 stalk celery with leaves*
*1 small bay leaf*
*1 teaspoon instant minced onion*
*½ teaspoon salt*
*½ cup Chicken Stock (see page 209) or Beef Stock (see page 209)*
*2 tablespoons pure maple syrup*
*½ teaspoon paprika*
*¼ cup unbleached flour or rice flour*

Preheat oven to 350°F

Prepare dry beans according to package directions. Drain. Combine beans, 3 cups water, parsley, celery, bay leaf, onion, and salt in a large saucepan. Bring to a boil. Simmer 2 hours. Beans should be mealy and tender.

Drain beans. Add stock, pure maple syrup, and paprika. Mix and bake for 15 minutes or until thoroughly heated. Make a paste of ½ cup water and flour and add as needed to thicken.

Are you a catsup freak? Here are two catsup recipes made without tomatoes. One substitutes rhubarb, the other beets and pumpkin! The spices overwhelm the taste of the fruit and vegetables to give the spicy catsup flavor.

**TOMATO-FREE CATSUP 1**

(No milk, egg, corn, wheat, rye, or citrus)
Makes 2 cups

*1 quart (4 cups) fresh or frozen (thawed) chopped rhubarb*
*½ cup water*
*¼ cup chopped onion or 1 tablespoon dried minced onion*
*½ cup honey*
*½ teaspoon salt*
*¼ cup allowed vinegar*
*¾ teaspoon cinnamon*
*½ teaspoon ginger*
*¼ teaspoon nutmeg*

Combine rhubarb, water, onion, honey, salt, and vinegar in a heavy 2-quart saucepan. Over medium heat, boil slowly until thick, stirring occasionally. Add spices, cook 5 more minutes. Cool. If too lumpy, put in blender until consistency is equivalent to that of tomato catsup. Refrigerate in a covered container.

**TOMATO-FREE CATSUP II**

(No milk, egg, corn, wheat, rye, or citrus)
Makes 3 cups

*1 8-ounce can sliced beets, undrained*
*⅔ cup allowed vinegar*
*⅓ cup water*
*½ cup pure maple syrup*
*¼ cup coarsely chopped onion*
*½ teaspoon cinnamon*

*½ teaspoon nutmeg*
*1 teaspoon salt*
*1 teaspoon Tabasco sauce*
*1 1-pound can pumpkin*

Combine all ingredients except pumpkin in a blender. Blend until smooth. Add pumpkin and mix thoroughly. Transfer to a medium-sized saucepan. Bring to a boil and simmer for 20 or 30 minutes. Cool and store in refrigerator.

### LASAGNA

(No egg, corn, rye, or citrus)
This lasagna recipe can use the Tomato-Free Spaghetti Sauce.
Serves 8

*6 cups allowed Tomato Spaghetti Sauce (see page 213) or Tomato-Free Spaghetti Sauce (see page 291)*
*8 ounces lasagna noodles (whole grain, if possible), cooked and drained*
*1 pound ricotta cheese or additive-free cottage cheese*
*8 ounces mozzarella cheese, shredded*
*1 cup grated Parmesan cheese*

Preheat oven to 350°F

Spread 2 cups spaghetti sauce in the bottom of 9 × 13-inch baking pan. Alternate layers of noodles, cheeses, and sauce, ending with mozzarella and Parmesan cheese on top. Bake for 50 minutes until bubbly. Remove from oven and let stand 10 minutes before serving.

## TOMATO-FREE PIZZA

(No egg, corn, rye, or citrus)

To ease those pizza hunger pangs, this tomato-free pizza should please.

Makes 2 12-inch pizzas

*1 recipe Pizza Crust (see page 211)*
*1 recipe Pesto Sauce (see below) or 2 cups Tomato-Free Spaghetti Sauce (see page 291)*
*½ pound ground beef*
*8 ounces mozzarella cheese, shredded*

Preheat oven to 350°F

Prepare pizza crust and sauce. Brown ground beef in a heavy skillet. Drain off excess grease. Add sauce and heat through. Spread sauce over pizza crust and top with cheese. Bake for 20 to 25 minutes until crust is lightly browned.

## PESTO SAUCE

(No egg, corn, wheat, rye, or citrus)

Here's another Italian sauce that can be used instead of tomato in a variety of dishes. Try it over spaghetti.

Makes ¾ cup

*2 to 4 tablespoons dried sweet basil*
*2 cloves garlic*
*½ cup grated Parmesan cheese*
*1 teaspoon salt*
*1 teaspoon black pepper*
*½ cup pure allowed vegetable oil*

Combine all dry ingredients in a blender. Add half the oil. Blend on high speed. Add remaining oil and blend until thoroughly mixed. Heat before serving. Refrigerate leftover sauce in a covered container.

### SPAGHETTI WITH CLAM SAUCE

(No milk, egg, corn, rye, or citrus)

Or top your spaghetti with a clam sauce instead of tomato.

Serves 4

*¾ pound spaghetti*
*½ cup chopped onion*
*1 clove garlic, minced*
*¼ cup pure allowed vegetable oil*
*2 8-ounce cans minced clams, reserving juice*
*½ cup dried parsley*
*1 teaspoon dried sweet basil*

Cook spaghetti according to package instructions. In a medium-sized skillet saute onion and garlic in oil until tender. Add the minced clams and their juice. Stir in parsley and basil. Heat through. Serve over spaghetti.

### TOMATO-FREE SPAGHETTI SAUCE

(No milk, egg, corn, wheat, rye, or citrus)

But what can be done for the tomato lover who has to have pizza, spaghetti, and lasagna? Try this spaghetti sauce.

Makes 4 cups

*1 15-ounce can beets*
*1 15-ounce can carrots*
*½ cup canned pumpkin*
*1 onion, quartered*
*3 cloves garlic*
*4 tablespoons allowed vinegar*
*2 teaspoons salt*
*1 teaspoon oregano*
*¼ cup unsweetened applesauce*

Put beets and carrots in blender with their juices and puree. Add pumpkin, onion, and garlic and continue to blend until smooth. Pour into a medium saucepan and add other ingredients. Bring to a boil and simmer for 20 to 30 minutes. Adjust seasonings to taste.

Now adapt some of your own favorite tomato recipes!

# APPENDIXES

# Notes

## 1: THE TRADITIONAL VIEW OF ALLERGIES

1. "Allergy: New Insights," *Newsweek* (Aug. 23, 1982), p. 40.
2. Kenneth P. Mathews, "Respiratory Atopic Disease," *Journal of the American Medical Association* (Vol. 248, No. 20, Nov. 1982), p. 2587.
3. "Allergy: New Insights," p. 40.
4. Rebecca H. Buckley and Kenneth P. Mathews, "Common 'Allergic' Skin Diseases," *Journal of the American Medical Association* (Vol. 248, No. 20, Nov. 1982), p. 2611.
5. Ibid., p. 2617.
6. "Respiratory Atopic Disease," p. 2587.
7. Roy Patterson and Martha Valentine, "Anaphylaxis and Related Emergencies Including Reactions Due to Insect Stings," *Journal of the American Medical Association* (Vol. 248, No. 20, Nov. 1982), p. 2632.

## 2: THE NONTRADITIONAL VIEW OF ALLERGIES

1. William G. Crook, "Food Allergy—The Great Masquerader," *Pediatric Clinics of North America* (Vol. 22, No. 1, Feb. 1975), pp. 227–238.
2. "A Doctors' Dispute," *Parade* (Aug. 1, 1982), p. 12.
3. Lawrence Dickey, Ed., *Clinical Ecology* (Springfield, Ill.: Thomas, 1970), pp. 310–320.
4. Theron Randolph and Ralph Moss, *An Alternative Approach to Allergies* (New York: Harper & Row, 1980), pp. 57–58.

5. William Duffy's *Sugar Blues* (Radnor, Penna.: Chilton, 1975) and Carlton Fredericks and Herman Goodman's *Low Blood Sugar and You* (New York: Grosset & Dunlap, 1969) discuss low blood sugar in detail.
6. Doris J. Rapp, *Allergies and the Hyperactive Child* (New York: Sovereign Books, 1979). See also William G. Crook, *Can Your Child Read? Is He Hyperactive?* (Jackson, Tenn.: Professional Books, 1975).
7. Randolph and Moss, *An Alternative Approach.* See also Marshall Mandell and Lynne Scanlon, *Dr. Mandell's 5-Day Allergy Relief System* (New York: Pocket Books, 1979).
8. William Philpott and Dwight K. Kalita, *Brain Allergies* (New Canaan, Conn.: Keats, 1980), pp. 117–118.
9. Roger J. Williams and Dwight K. Kalita, eds., *A Physician's Handbook on Orthomolecular Medicine* (New York: Pergamon Press, 1977), pp. 156–160.
10. Alexander Schauss, *Diet, Crime and Delinquency* (Berkeley: Parker House, 1980).

## 8: HEREDITY AND INFANT FEEDING PRACTICES—AN OUNCE OF PREVENTION

1. Claude A. Frazier, *Coping with Food Allergy* (New York: Quadrangle/New York Times, 1975), p. 4.
2. John W. Gerrard, *Food Allergy: New Perspectives* (Springfield, Ill.: Thomas, 1980), pp. 209–218.
3. Lendon H. Smith, *Improving Your Child's Behavior Chemistry* (Englewood Cliffs, N.J.: Prentice-Hall, 1976).
4. "Feeding a Baby with Allergies," *Allergy Information Newsletter* (March 1972), pp. 1–2.
5. Ibid., p. 2.

## 9: CANDIDA ALBICANS: A BEASTLY YEAST

1. C. Orian Truss, "The Role of Candida Albicans in Human Illness," *Journal of Orthomolecular Psychiatry* (Vol. 10, No. 4, 1981), pp. 228–238.
2. C. Orian Truss, "Tissue Injury Induced by Candida Albicans: Mental and Neurological Manifestations," *Journal of Orthomolecular Psychiatry* (Vol. 7, No. 1, 1978), pp. 18–19.
3. Ibid.

4. William G. Crook, *The Yeast Connection* (Jackson, Tenn.: Professional Books, 1983).
5. See C. Orian Truss, *The Missing Diagnosis* (Birmingham, Ala.: Truss, 1983).
6. C. Orian Truss, "Restoration of Immunologic Competence to Candida Albicans," *Journal of Orthomolecular Psychiatry* (Vol. 9, No. 4, 1980), pp. 289–300.
7. William G. Crook, "About Yeast Infection: Candida Albicans or Monilia" (unpublished).
8. Truss, *Missing Diagnosis*, pp. 144–146.
9. An excellent conference devoted to Candida albicans was held in Dallas in 1982, with Dr. Truss and other interested doctors. Tapes of this meeting are available from: Creative Audio, 8751 Osborne, Highland, Ind. 46322.

## 10: IMPROVING YOUR DIET

1. *Dietary Goals for the United States*, prepared by staff of Select Committee on Nutrition and Human Needs, United States Senate (Dec. 1977), pp. 73–74.
2. Reader's Digest, *Eat Better, Live Better* (Pleasantville, N.Y.: Reader's Digest, 1982), p. 16.
3. Michael F. Jacobson, *Nutrition Scoreboard* (New York: Avon Books, 1974), p. 46.
4. Reader's Digest, *Eat Better*, p. 17.
5. Hal A. Huggins, *Why Raise Ugly Kids?* (Westport, Conn.: Arlington House, 1981), p. 141.
6. Ibid., pp. 146–147.
7. Reader's Digest, *Eat Better*, p. 371.
8. Huggins, *Why Raise Ugly Kids?*, pp. 141–149.

## 11: OVERCOMING NUTRITIONAL DEFICIENCIES

1. "What's Missing in Your Diet," *Good Housekeeping* (Jan. 1983), pp. 164–166.
2. Hal A. Huggins, *Why Raise Ugly Kids?* (Westport, Conn.: Arlington House, 1981), p. 124.
3. Unless otherwise noted all food values in this chapter are from *Nutrition Almanac* (New York: McGraw-Hill, 1973, 1975), pp. 186–219.

4. Hal A. Huggins, *How to Balance the Chemistry of the Periodontal Patient* (Colorado Springs: HAH Publications, 1981), pp. 12–13.
5. These figures are from: Carl C. Pfeiffer, *Mental and Emotional Nutrients* (New Canaan, Conn.: Keats, 1975), pp. 241–242.
6. Ibid., pp. 256–257.
7. Donald O. Rudin, "The Dominant Diseases of Modernized Societies as Omega-3 Essential Fatty Acid Deficiency Syndrome: Substrate Beriberi," *Medical Hypotheses* (Vol. 8, 1982), pp. 17–47.
8. Donald O. Rudin, "Protocol for Essential Fatty Acid Deficiency Study" (July 8, 1981, unpublished).
9. Richard A. Passwater, *Evening Primrose Oil* (New Canaan, Conn.: Keats, 1981), pp. 1–30.
10. Jonathon V. Wright, *Dr. Wright's Book of Nutritional Therapy* (Emmaus, Penna.: Rodale Press, 1979), pp. 387–392.

## 12: LIMITING YOUR EXPOSURE TO TOXIC METALS

1. Carl C. Pfeiffer, *Mental and Elemental Nutrients* (New Canaan, Conn.: Keats, 1975), pp. 317–321.
2. "The 24 Hour Mercury Hypersensitivity Patch Test," *Momentum Newsletter* (No. 2, Nov. 1982), p. 4 (published by Toxic Element Research Foundation).
3. "Why Complacency," *Momentum Newsletter* (No. 2, Nov. 1982), p. 1.
4. Hal A. Huggins, "Mercury: A Factor in Mental Illness," *Journal of Orthomolecular Psychiatry* (Vol. 11, No. 1, 1982), pp. 3–16.
5. "Mercury Testing Protocol Developed by Dr. Hal A. Huggins," *Momentum Newsletter* (No. 1, 1982), p. 2.
6. Mercury patch test is available to your doctor or dentist from: Tox Supply, PO Box 546, Colorado Springs, Colorado 80901.
7. "What Does the Hair Mecury Level Mean?," *Momentum Newsletter* (No. 2, Nov. 1982), p. 3.
8. "Mercury Testing Protocol," p. 2.
9. Mercury vapor can be measured by a Bacharach Mercury Sniffer, available from: United Technologies Bacharach, 5100 Patrick Henry Drive, Santa Clara, California 95050.
10. "Protecting the Mercury Hypersensitive Patient During Amalgam Removal," *Momentum Newsletter* (No. 2, Nov. 1982), p. 5.

11. Pfeiffer, *Mental and Elemental Nutrients*, pp. 311–317. See also: Michael Lesser, *Vitamin and Mineral Therapy* (New York: Grove Press, 1980), pp. 154–160, and Alexander Schauss, *Diet, Crime and Delinquency* (Berkeley: Parker House, 1980), pp. 32–45.
12. Pfeiffer, pp. 304–307; Lesser, pp. 162–164.
13. Pfeiffer, pp. 321–323; Lesser, p. 165.
14. Pfeiffer, pp. 325–340; Lesser, pp. 133–136.

## 13: REDUCING STRESS IN YOUR LIFE

1. Mildred Carter, *Helping Yourself with Foot Reflexology* (West Nyack, N.Y.: Parker House, 1969).

# APPENDIX A

# Sample Common Foods Elimination Diet

These sample menus and hypothetical diet diary should give you a good idea of how to pursue the Common Foods Elimination Diet. Remember that milk, eggs, corn, wheat, chocolate, rye, citrus, and sugar, as well as artificial colorings, flavorings, and perservatives, are avoided in all forms for a week, or until you feel better for several days. Then, one day at a time, each food is reintroduced and mental and physical symptoms are noted.

For the *italicized* items under foods, you will find recipes elsewhere in this book. Use the Recipe Index to locate them. On food items followed by two asterisks (**), double the recipe, reserving leftovers for another meal or snack.

*Sample Common Foods Elimination Diet*

## DAY 1

| *Meal* | *Foods* | *Diary of Reactions* |
|---|---|---|
| BREAKFAST | Hamburger or chopped steak (no bun) or *sausage patties*<br>Fried potatoes (in pure safflower oil)<br>Unsweetened applesauce<br>Unsweetened pineapple juice or tomato juice | Tired, draggy all morning. |
| SNACK | Apple or pear (peel if waxed) | |
| LUNCH | Plain hamburger with *tomato catsup*<br>Allowed potato chips (no preservatives, fried in pure safflower oil)<br>Unsweetened allowed fruit<br>Carrot sticks<br>Unsweetened grape juice | Irritable. I miss my favorite foods already. |
| SNACK | Shelled peanuts, carrots, celery | |
| DINNER | *Fried chicken***<br>Potatoes or rice<br>Peas<br>Tossed salad with allowed dressing<br>Allowed fruit | Really depressed tonight. How will I survive another week? I HATE this diet. |
| SNACK | Rice cakes with natural peanut butter | |

## DAY 2

| | | |
|---|---|---|
| BREAKFAST | Oatmeal with pure honey or pure maple syrup, or *oat or rice pancakes*<br>Broiled pork chops<br>Pears or peaches (fresh or water-packed)<br>Unsweetened pineapple juice or grape juice | Down, depressed, aching. Slept poorly all night. |
| SNACK | Raw almonds, grape juice | |
| LUNCH | Cold leftover *fried chicken*<br>Allowed potato chips<br>Fresh grapes<br>Several dates<br>Ice water | In tears all morning. |
| SNACK | Natural peanut butter on celery<br>Unsweetened apple juice | |
| DINNER | *Tomato spaghetti sauce* on rice<br>Lettuce salad with allowed dressing<br>Green beans with allowed safflower margarine<br>*Fruit ice* or melon in season<br>Ice water | Very achy, depressed tonight. Miss wheat especially. |
| SNACK | Peanuts or walnuts | |

## DAY 3

| | | |
|---|---|---|
| BREAKFAST | Hamburger or *sausage patties*<br>Oatmeal with pure honey or maple syrup<br>Banana or fresh peach<br>Unsweetened pineapple juice or allowed herb tea | Slightly better night. Would give anything for eggs this morning. |
| SNACK | Celery with peanut butter | |
| LUNCH | Tuna or chicken salad with *egg-free mayonnaise***<br>*Pumpkin bread* or rice cakes<br>Carrot sticks<br>Raw apple or pear (unwaxed)<br>Tomato juice or ice water | Better morning. Not so tired. |
| SNACK | Cold leftover *fried chicken* | |
| DINNER | Fish (baked or broiled)<br>Baked or sweet potato<br>Asparagus or green beans<br>Fruit cup of allowed fruits<br>*Maple apple pudding*<br>Unsweetened pineapple juice or herb tea | Achy but better mentally. |
| SNACK | Unsweetened pineapple chunks or strawberries<br>Peanuts, cashews, or walnuts | |

## DAY 4

| Meal | Foods | Notes |
| --- | --- | --- |
| BREAKFAST | Lamb chop or hamburger<br>*Pumpkin bread* or rice cakes with allowed jam<br>Unsweetened applesauce<br>Apple juice or ice water | Slept well, aching much better, feel energetic. |
| SNACK | Peanuts, walnuts, sunflower seeds<br>Allowed fruit | |
| LUNCH | Leftover tuna or chicken salad on rice cakes or lettuce<br>Carrots, celery<br>Peaches (fresh or water packed)<br>*Pumpkin bread* with allowed margarine<br>Grape juice or ice water | Excellent morning. |
| SNACK | Peanut butter and allowed jam on rice cakes | |
| DINNER | Beef stew thickened with allowed starch<br>Rice<br>*Pumpkin cookies* or allowed fresh fruit<br>Ice water or herb tea | Haven't felt so great in years. |
| SNACK | *Pumpkin cookies*<br>Peanut butter on celery or rice cakes<br>Unsweetened allowed juice | |

## DAY 5

Repeat menus for Day 1

Great all day. Sinus drippage seems to be stopping.

## DAY 6

Repeat menus for Day 2

Good day.

## DAY 7

Repeat menus for Day 3 or Day 2

I'm doing so well I'm scared to reintroduce the foods starting tomorrow.

## DAY 8—Reintroduce Eggs

| | | |
|---|---|---|
| BREAKFAST | Scrambled eggs (omit milk, scramble in a little safflower oil)<br>Fried potatoes<br>Unsweetened applesauce<br>Unsweetened pineapple juice | Legs ache after breakfast. Eggs? |
| SNACK | Apple or pear (unwaxed), hard-boiled egg | Feel HORRIBLE. Legs ache, depressed. STOP SERVING EGGS. |
| LUNCH | Plain hamburger with *tomato catsup*<br>Allowed potato chips<br>Carrot sticks<br>Unsweetened allowed fruit<br>Ice water | |
| SNACK | Shelled peanuts, carrots, celery | |
| DINNER | *Fried chicken***<br>Potatoes or rice<br>Peas or broccoli<br>Tossed salad with allowed dressing<br>Allowed fruit | Still dragging. |
| SNACK | Rice cakes with natural peanut butter | Feeling better tonight. |

## DAY 9—Reintroduce Sugar

| | | |
|---|---|---|
| BREAKFAST | Oatmeal with sugar<br>Broiled pork chops<br>Peaches with sugar<br>Sweetened pineapple juice (with sugar) | Seem okay this morning so will try sugar. Surprisingly, I don't even want it. |
| SNACK | Raw almonds, grape juice with sugar added | Hard to concentrate, sleepy. |
| LUNCH | Sugar cubes<br>Cold leftover *fried chicken*<br>Fresh grapes<br>Several dates<br>Ice water | |
| SNACK | Natural peanut butter on celery<br>Apple juice | Bad headache. Definitely worse on sugar. STOP SERVING SUGAR. |
| DINNER | *Tomato spaghetti sauce* on rice<br>Lettuce salad with allowed dressing<br>Green beans with allowed margarine<br>*Fruit ice* or melon in season<br>Ice water | |
| SNACK | Peanuts or walnuts | Reaction seems over. Just more tired. |

## DAY 10—Reintroduce Corn

| | | |
|---|---|---|
| BREAKFAST | Corn-on-the-cob with allowed margarine<br>*Sausage patties*<br>Banana or fresh allowed fruit<br>Unsweetened pineapple juice | Seem okay this morning. |
| SNACK | Popcorn popped in safflower oil | Okay. |
| LUNCH | Popcorn<br>Cold leftover *fried chicken*<br>*Pumpkin bread*<br>Carrot sticks<br>Raw apple or pear (unwaxed)<br>Tomato juice | |
| SNACK | Popcorn<br>Celery with natural peanut butter | Okay. |
| DINNER | Corn-on-the-cob with allowed margarine<br>Fish (baked or broiled)<br>Asparagus or green beans<br>Allowed fruits in a fruit cup<br>*Pumpkin cookies*<br>Tomato juice | Darn. Nose is streaming. |
| SNACK | Popcorn | Nose is still streaming. Nausea, stomachache. STOP CORN. |

## DAY 11—Reintroduce Wheat

| | | |
|---|---|---|
| BREAKFAST | Wholewheat pancakes (no milk, sugar, or eggs) with pure maple syrup and allowed margarine or cream-of-wheat cereal (no milk or sugar)<br>Lamb chop or hamburger<br>Apple juice<br>Grapes | Okay this morning. |
| SNACK | Leftover pancake or spread banana with natural peanut butter and roll in honey, wheat germ, and coconut (unsweetened) | |
| LUNCH | Tuna or chicken salad made with *egg-free mayonnaise* on rice cakes or lettuce<br>Peaches (fresh or water-packed)<br>*Pumpkin bread* with allowed margarine<br>Grape juice | Dark circles are back. Much more depressed. Legs ache. Nose stuffy. STOP WHEAT. |
| SNACK | Banana, allowed nuts | |
| DINNER | Beef stew<br>Rice<br>*Pumpkin cookies* or allowed fruit<br>Ice water or herb tea | |
| SNACK | *Pumpkin cookies*<br>Peanut butter on celery or rice cakes | |

## DAY 12—Reintroduce Rye

| | | |
|---|---|---|
| BREAKFAST | Natural rye crackers with allowed margarine and jam<br>Hamburger or *sausage patties*<br>Fried potatoes in pure safflower oil<br>Unsweetened applesauce<br>Water or herb tea | Okay this morning. |
| SNACK | Natural rye crackers with natural peanut butter | |
| LUNCH | Natural rye crackers with allowed margarine and jam<br>Plain hamburger with *tomato catsup*<br>Allowed potato chips<br>Carrot sticks<br>Tomato juice | Feel fine. |
| SNACK | Natural rye crackers with peanut butter<br>Carrots, celery | |
| DINNER | *Fried chicken***<br>Baked potatoes<br>Peas or broccoli<br>Tossed salad with allowed dressing<br>Natural rye cracker with allowed margarine<br>Fruit in season | Doing well. Keeping fingers crossed. |
| SNACK | Natural rye cracker with peanut butter | Good day. Not sensitive to rye. Hooray! |

## DAY 13—Reintroduce Citrus

| | | |
|---|---|---|
| BREAKFAST | Oatmeal with honey or pure maple syrup<br>Broiled pork chops<br>Fresh orange sections<br>Unsweetened pineapple juice | I only like oranges so will just reintroduce these. |
| SNACK | Fresh-squeezed orange juice<br>Allowed nuts or cold leftover *fried chicken* | |
| LUNCH | Cold leftover *fried chicken*<br>Allowed potato chips<br>Fresh orange sections<br>Unsweetened pineapple juice | Fine so far. |
| SNACK | Fresh-squeezed orange juice<br>Peanut butter on celery | |
| DINNER | *Tomato spaghetti sauce* on rice<br>Fruit salad with fresh orange sections<br>Green beans with allowed margarine<br>*Fruit ice* or unsweetened pineapple chunks<br>Ice water | Good day so far. |
| SNACK | Fresh orange sections | Hooray again! I feel good. |

## DAY 14—Reintroduce Chocolate

| | | |
|---|---|---|
| BREAKFAST | *Sausage patties*<br>*Oat or rice pancakes*<br>Banana or fresh peach<br>Unsweetened pineapple juice<br>Piece of unsweetened chocolate | Okay this morning. |
| SNACK | Rice cake with peanut butter<br>Piece of unsweetened chocolate | After snack, nose is streaming. Mad at the world, can't concentrate. STOP CHOCOLATE. |
| LUNCH | Leftover cold *fried chicken*<br>*Pumpkin bread*<br>Carrot sticks<br>Raw apple or pear (unwaxed)<br>Tomato juice | |
| SNACK | Pineapple chunks (unsweetened) or grapes<br>Allowed nuts | |
| DINNER | Fish (baked or broiled)<br>Baked potato or sweet potato<br>Asparagus or green beans<br>*Fruit ice* | |
| SNACK | Peanuts, cashews, or walnuts | Still grumpy tonight. |

## DAY 15—Reintroduce Food Colorings

| | | |
|---|---|---|
| BREAKFAST | Lamb chop or hamburger<br>*Pumpkin bread*<br>Unsweetened applesauce<br>All food colorings mixed together and ½ teaspoon added to grape juice or ice water | Okay this morning.<br>After drinking colored water, I feel really hyper. Can't sit still, can't concentrate. Joints ache. STOP COLORS. |
| SNACK | *Pumpkin bread* or rice cakes | |
| LUNCH | Tuna or chicken salad on rice cakes or lettuce<br>Carrots, celery<br>*Pumpkin bread*<br>Grapes<br>Ice water | |
| SNACK | Leftover cold *fried chicken*<br>Carrots, celery, cherry tomatoes | |
| DINNER | Beef stew<br>Rice<br>*Pumpkin cookies* or allowed fresh fruit<br>Unsweetened allowed juice or herb tea | Tired, depressed, crying. |
| SNACK | Peanut butter on rice cakes or celery | |

## DAY 16—Reintroduce Milk

| | | |
|---|---|---|
| BREAKFAST | Hamburger or *sausage patties*<br>Fried potatoes (in pure safflower oil)<br>Unsweetened applesauce<br>Glass of milk | Hooray! Last day. Feel okay this morning. |
| SNACK | Glass of milk<br>*Pumpkin cookie* or allowed nuts | Tired this morning? |
| LUNCH | Glass of milk<br>Plain hamburger with *tomato catsup*<br>Allowed potato chips<br>Grapes | Pooped. From colors yesterday or milk today? |
| SNACK | Glass of milk<br>Peanut butter on rice cakes | |
| DINNER | Glass of milk<br>*Fried chicken*<br>Peas with uncolored butter<br>Baked potato with uncolored butter<br>*Fruit ice*<br>Cooked carrots with uncolored butter | Tired. |
| SNACK | *Pumpkin bread* or rice cakes with peanut butter or uncolored butter | Can't keep awake. Nose is stuffy. Legs ache. Milk must be a problem. STOP MILK. |

# APPENDIX B

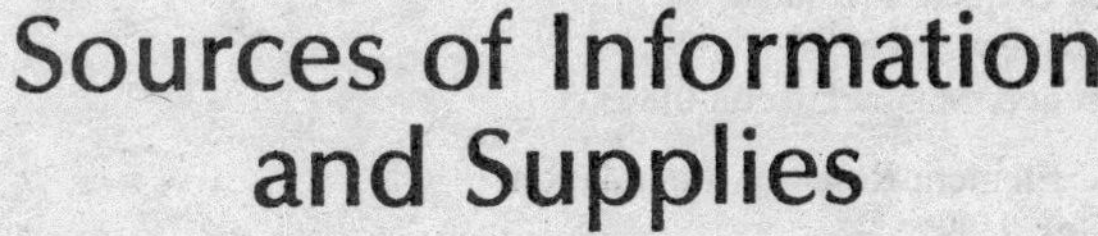

# Sources of Information and Supplies

## AIR FILTERS

Dome Laboratories
Division of Miles Laboratories, Inc.
400 Morgan Lane
West Haven, Connecticut 06516

## COTTON PRODUCTS

Ecologist's Cotton Co-op
2986 Talisman Drive
Dallas, Texas 75229

## DOCTORS AND DENTISTS

The following groups will provide a list of members (doctors and dentists) who are interested in allergy, orthomolecular medicine, and nutrition and may be practicing near you.

American Academy of Otolaryngic Allergy
1101 Vermont Avenue, N.W., Suite 302
Washington, D.C. 20005

International Academy of Preventive Medicine
10409 Town and Country Way, Suite 200
Houston, Texas 77024

Orthomolecular Medical Society
2698 Pacific Avenue
San Francisco, California 94115

Society for Clinical Ecology
James O'Shea, President
50 Prospect Street
Lawrence, Massachusetts 01843

Toxic Element Research Foundation
PO Box 2589
Colorado Springs, Colorado 80901

*The following physicians practice clinical ecology in either a controlled environmental hospital unit or isolated rooms:*

Thurman Bullock, Jr., M.D., and Francis Carroll, M.D.
722 North Brown Street
Chadbourn, North Carolina 28431

Marshall Mandell, M.D.
The New England Foundation for Allergic and Environmental Diseases
3 Brush Street
Norwalk, Connecticut 06850

Theron Randolph, M.D., and Robert Marshall, M.D.
505 North Lake Shore Drive
Chicago, Illinois 60611

William Rea, M.D., and Ralph E. Smiley, M.D.
8345 Walnut Hill Lane, Suite 240
Dallas, Texas 75231

John Selner, M.D., and Kendall Gerdes, M.D.
Presbyterian Hospital
1719 East 19th Avenue
Denver, Colorado 80218

**FOODS**

Czimer Foods, Inc.
RR #1, Box 285
Lockport, Illinois 60441
(Exotic meats.)

Walnut Acres
Penns Creek, Pennsylvania 17862
(Wide assortment of organic foods.)

### FORMALDEHYDE TEST KIT

S. A. Rogers, M.D.
2800 West Genesee Street
Syracuse, New York 13219

### HAIR ANALYSIS

Body-Chem, Inc.
P.O. Box 2589
Colorado Springs, Colorado 80906

Doctor's Data
30 West 101 Roosevelt Road
PO Box 397
West Chicago, Illinois 60185

Mineralab, Inc.
PO Box 5012
Hayward, California 94540

### INFORMATION AND NEWSLETTERS

Academy of Orthomolecular Psychiatry
1691 Northern Boulevard
Manhasset, New York 10030

Allergy Information Association
25 Poynter Drive, Room 7
Weston, Ontario, Canada M9R 1K8
(The Allergy Information Association is a superb volunteer organization dedicated to helping allergy sufferers. They publish an excellent newsletter, pamphlets on different topics, and a cookbook.)

Biofeedback Society of America
University of Colorado Medical College C268
4200 East Ninth Avenue
Denver, Colorado 80262

Center for Science in the Public Interest (CSPI)
1775 S Street NW
Washington, D.C. 20009
(The goal of CSPI is to improve the quality of American diets through research and public education. They publish *Nutrition Action Magazine* and have several excellent posters available.)

Clinical Ecology
109 West Olive
Fort Collins, Colorado 80524
(They are publishing a new medical journal, *Clinical Ecology: Archives of the Society for Clinical Ecology.)*

Feingold Association of United States
Drawer A-G
Holtsville, New York 11742
(The Feingold Association is a volunteer group of parents dedicated to helping other parents of hyperactive and learning-disabled children through a newsletter, *Pure Facts*, and local Feingold support groups.)

Healthful Living Company
Eileen Yoder, Director
PO Box 563
Goshen, Indiana 46526
(*The Food Allergy and Nutrition Newsletter* focuses on advice and recipes for allergics.)

Human Ecology Action League (HEAL)
505 North Lake Shore Drive
Chicago, Illinois 60611
(HEAL is very concerned about the effect of the environment on health. Their superb newsletter, *The Human Ecologist,* discusses various topics in clinical ecology. They have chapters in many other states which act as support groups for the members.)

The Huxley Institute for Biosocial Research
1114 First Avenue
New York, New York 10021
(The Huxley Institute is concerned with educating the public and professionals about the biochemical causes of mental illness. They have many excellent tapes and reprints available.)

La Leche League International, Inc.
9616 Minneapolis Avenue
Franklin Park, Illinois 60131
(La Leche League is a nonprofit organization dedicated to good mothering through breast-feeding. Local groups offer information, books, support, and encouragement for nursing mothers.)

New York Institute for Child Development
205 Lexington Avenue
New York, New York 10016
(The New York Institute for Child Development publishes an informative newsletter, *Reaching Children*, about diet, behavior, and learning disabilities. They have some fascinating cassette tapes available.)

Prevention Magazine
33 East Minor Street
Emmaus, Pennsylvania 18049
(*Prevention* magazine is a monthly publication devoted to better health through proper diet.)

Toxic Element Research Foundation (TERF)
PO Box 2589
Colorado Springs, Colorado 80901
(TERF publishes an interesting newsletter about the effects of toxic metals, especially mercury.)

## MASKS

Human Ecology Research Foundation of the Southwest
12110 Webbs Chapel, Suite 305E
Dallas, Texas 75234
(Cotton mask with charcoal filter screens chemicals, dust, and pollens.)

## PEST CONTROL

Human Ecology Research Foundation of the Southwest
12110 Webbs Chapel, Suite 305E
Dallas, Texas 75234
(Ultra-Sonic Pest Control Unit emits ultra-high-intensity sound waves that repel insects and pests.)

## VACUUM CLEANER

Rainbow-Rexair Vacuum Sales and Service
605 Spring Lake Drive
Bedford, Texas 76021

## VITAMINS AND MINERALS

Bronsons Pharmaceuticals
4526 Rinetti Lane
LaCanada, California 91011
(Will supply complete list of filters in their products, on request.)

Matrix Minerals
PO Box 546
Colorado Springs, Colorado 80906
(Compounds its minerals with several agents—proteinates, chelates, ascorbates, citrates—to enhance absorption.)

Nutricology
2336-C Stanwell Circle
Concord, California 94520
(Products especially made for people with allergies. Sources for vitamins and minerals are carefully chosen to avoid allergenic substances, and the vitamins and minerals are compounded to provide allergy relief. Nutricology also publishes an interesting newsletter.)

Willner Chemists
330 Lexington Avenue
New York, New York 10016

## WATER PURIFIERS AND DISTILLERS

Puro Filter Corporation of America
56-45 58th Street
Maspeth, New York 11378

Pure Water, Inc.
3725 Towzalin Avenue
Lincoln, Nebraska 68505

Durastill of Atlanta
6321 Hunting Creek Road
Atlanta, Georgia 30328

# APPENDIX C

# Common Food Additives and Contaminants

## FOOD ADDITIVES

**ARTIFICIAL COLORINGS:** Some of the common artificial colors are:

—Blue No. 1 (Brilliant blue)
—Blue No. 2 (Indigotine)
—Citrus Red No. 2
—Green No. 3 (Fast green)
—Orange B
—Red No. 3 (Erythrosine)
—Red No. 40 (Allura)
—Yellow No. 5 (Tartrazine)
—Yellow No. 6 (Sunset yellow)

These dyes are derived from processing coal. Many researchers believe they are poorly tested for safety. They may lead to hyperactivity, seizures, depression, hives, or arthritis in the sensitive person. Often labels only state, "U.S. certified color added" or "artificial color"; they do not specify which dye is present. Butter, ice cream, and cheese may be dyed without stating that information. Artificial colorings in drugs may also cause severe problems for unsuspecting, chemically sensitive people. An allergy to one color does not necessarily mean an allergy to all of them.

**ARTIFICIAL FLAVORINGS:** This group of compounds is used to flavor foods. Dozens of chemicals may be required to imitate one flavor so it's even harder to track down offending components. These flavorings are frequently found with artificial colorings and sugar. Choose products with natural flavors. Then if a reaction occurs, you'll know what food you're dealing with.

**BHA AND BHT:** These abbreviations stand for butylated hydroxyanisole and butylated hydroxytoluene, respectively. These chemicals are widely used as preservatives to prolong the shelf life of nuts, beverages, cereals, oils, and snack foods. They may be present in some oils without appearing on the label if the oils were purchased by the manufacturer with the preservatives already added. They cause some sensitive children to become hyperactive and may lead to other allergic reactions in susceptible people. These chemicals are believed by some researchers to be poorly tested for safety.

**CAFFEINE:** This stimulant is added to soft drinks and occurs naturally in coffee, tea, and cocoa. It disrupts normal blood sugar levels in sensitive individuals. Some people are allergic to the caffeine itself. It may cause withdrawal symptoms when removed suddenly from the diet.

**CALCIUM PROPIONATE:** This chemical is used to inhibit mold growth and occurs naturally in some foods. Allergic reactions have been reported.

**CARAMEL COLOR:** This color may be derived from heat-treating one of the following: sucrose (cane or beets), dextrose or glucose from corn, molasses, and lactose (milk sugar). Or caramel color may be artificial.

**CASEIN OR SODIUM CASEINATE:** Casein is the protein in milk and may cause problems for milk-sensitive people. It's used as a thickening and whitening agent.

**CITRIC ACID:** This chemical occurs widely in nature. Commercially it is usually made from corn or sugar beet molasses but may also be produced from lemon or pineapple. Some individuals are sensitive to citric acid whether it occurs naturally or is made artificially. In addition to foods, some over-the-counter medications contain citric acid.

**EDTA:** This abbreviation stands for ethylene diamine tetraacetic acid. Used to trap metal impurities acquired during processing of foods, EDTA appears to be safe. It is widely found in salad dressings, mayonnaise, processed fruits and vegetables, and soft drinks—

to name just a few. EDTA is also used by doctors for medical purposes.

**EXTENDERS:** These foods are added as fillers because they are usually less expensive than the major ingredient in the product. Soy, starch, glucose, breading, or milk casein may be used. Unless the label lists specific information, you won't know which one is present.

**FOOD STARCH OR MODIFIED FOOD STARCH:** This may be derived from wheat, corn, sorghum, arrowroot, tapioca, or potatoes.

**LECITHIN:** This nutritious chemical is found widely in nature. Food processors use it as an antioxidant and emulsifier. Soybean is the most common source by far for lecithin used by the food industry.

**MALT:** This may be processed from yeast-fermented corn, wheat, or barley.

**MONOSODIUM GLUTAMATE (MSG):** This chemical is very widely used in soups, poultry, cheese, sauces, and the like as a flavor-enhancer, although it is no longer added to baby foods. It is known to cause the "Chinese Restaurant Syndrome" (severe headache) in sensitive people. It used to be extracted from soybean or seaweed but is now also derived from wheat, corn, or sugar beets.

**NATURAL DYES:** Here are some vegetable dyes commonly used for coloring that seem preferable to coal tar dyes, although they may cause problems in sensitive people:

—Annatto (from seeds of annatto tree)
—Paprika (dried pod of sweet pepper)
—Tumeric (dried herb)
—Saffron (dried plant)
—Grape (grape skins)
—Dehydrated beets
—Riboflavin (synthetic or natural)
—Carrot oil (carrots)
—Beta-carotene (synthetic or natural)

**NATURAL GUMS:** Karaya, arabic (acacia), and tragacanth are members of the legume family and are known to cause allergic reactions in some people. Other gums you may encounter are locust bean (carob), chicle (chewing gum), guar, ghatti, and carrageen. These gums are used as thickening agents and stabilizers. Some researchers feel they have been poorly tested for safety.

**POTASSIUM IODATE OR POTASSIUM IODIDE:** This chemical is added to salt to provide iodine, a necessary nutrient. It may bother some sensitive people.

**QUININE:** This flavoring agent is used in beverages and can cause reactions in sensitive people.

**SODIUM BENZOATE:** This chemical is used as a preservative. It occurs naturally, but persons sensitive to aspirin and salicylates may also be sensitive to sodium benzoate.

**SODIUM CHLORIDE:** This is common table salt. A diet too high in sodium may contribute to high blood pressure.

**SODIUM NITRITE AND SODIUM NITRATES:** These chemicals are widely used in ham, bacon, hot dogs, smoked fish, and luncheon meats as preservatives and color-stabilizers. They are no longer added to baby foods. They have recently come under attack as cancer-causing agents and may cause joint inflammation, severe headaches, and other reactions in sensitive people.

**SULFUR DIOXIDE OR SODIUM BISULFITE:** These chemicals prevent discoloration of dried fruit and inhibit the growth of bacteria. Dried fruits without sulfur dioxide are available and just as tasty, even though they look brown and discolored. French fries are also dipped in sulfur dioxide to prevent discoloration. Fresh asparagus may be treated with sulfur dioxide to improve the color. Corn is soaked in sulfur dioxide at the beginning of its processing into corn products. Some doctors have found sulfur to be a major contaminant in our food supply causing acute mental and physical symptoms.

**SWEETENERS:** Many different types of sweeteners are used. Here are some of the most common:

1. *Aspartame*—a new low-calorie sweetener made from two amino acids. In the body it is processed as a natural, nutritive food.

Although it underwent vigorous safety testing before the Food and Drug Administration approved its use, how it will be tolerated by sensitive allergic people remains to be seen. Because it is cut with milk sugar, it may bother those sensitive to milk. Aspartame should also be avoided by people with phenylketonuria, who must restrict their intake of protein foods that contain phenylalanine (one of the amino acids in aspartame).

2. *Corn syrup*—a sweet liquid made from cornstarch. Those sensitive to corn are usually sensitive to corn syrup.
3. *Cyclamate*—an artificial sweetener banned by the Food and Drug Administration because it is suspected of causing cancer.
4. *Dextrose* or *glucose*—one of the most common compounds found in living organisms. But sensitive people may react to dextrose used as an additive if they are allergic to the plant from which the dextrose was made. Corn is a common source.
5. *Mannitol*—a sweetening agent used in low-calorie foods because the body can use only half its calories. Mannitol is also used in noncariogenic chewing gum (sugarless) because it does not promote tooth decay. It is synthesized from sugar.
6. *Saccharin*—a widely used artificial sweetener. Products containing saccharin must now carry a warning label because saccharin is suspected of causing cancer. Sensitive people may react adversely to saccharin.
7. *Sorbitol*—a sweetener related to sugar and mannitol and containing as many calories. Because sorbitol is absorbed slowly into the bloodstream, blood sugar levels elevate only slightly, making it a useful sweetener for diabetics. Sorbitol is also relatively noncariogenic.
8. *Sucrose*—ordinary table sugar, usually derived from sugar cane or beets. Sucrose promotes tooth decay, affects blood sugar levels, and encourages yeast growth in the Candida-sensitive person. It may also cause reactions in those who are sensitive to the source of the sugar.

**VITAMINS AND MINERALS:** These chemicals may be added for nutritional reasons or because they perform some other function. They may be either natural or synthetic. Some individuals may be sensitive to one or both forms. Commonly found as additivies are:

—Alpha-tocopherol (vitamin E; prevents oils from becoming rancid).

—Beta-carotene (precursor for vitamin A; used for nutrition and as a coloring agent).
—Ascorbic acid (vitamin C; used as a color-stabilizer and antioxidant; sodium ascorbate is a more soluble form).
—Ferrous gluconate (an iron compound; used for nutriton and as a coloring agent).
—Ergosterol (a natural steroid converted by ultraviolet radiation to vitamin D; mostly from yeast).
—Niacin, riboflavin, and thiamine (B vitamins; often from brewer's yeast and rice).

## UNLISTED CHEMICAL CONTAMINANTS

**ANTIBIOTICS, HORMONES, AND TRANQUILIZERS:** Meat, poultry, and fish may contain traces of these chemicals in sufficient quantity to bother susceptible people. Antibiotics are used to keep the animals healthy, and antibiotic solutions may be applied after the animal is slaughtered to prevent spoilage. Hormones are used to increase the animals' bulk and to shorten the time until market. Animals may be injected with tranquilizers prior to slaughter.

**BLEACHING AGENTS:** The bleaching agents used to whiten flour can cause reactions in susceptible people. Buy unbleached flour or, better yet, wholewheat flour.

**FUMIGANTS:** Methyl bromide is a fumigant that must be used (Federal law) on dates and other dried fruits that are shipped across state lines. Nuts, dry peas, beans, and lentils are also fumigated.

**FUNGICIDES:** Fungicides are used on packing crates for vegetables and fruits to prevent mold growth. But the vapors contaminate the fruits and vegetables.

**GAS FUMES:** Fruits ripen because of their natural production of ethylene gas. But many fruits are picked unripened and then gassed with natural or synthetic ethylene, causing problems for the susceptible person. Bananas are a common example. If you sometimes tolerate bananas but not on other occasions, it may be because of the presence of ethylene gas.

Gas-roasted coffee is another common problem since just about all commercial coffee is processed this way. If you're sensitive to coffee, it may be the gas fumes, not the coffee itself. Sugar (cane, beet, and corn) also has a processing step when it's exposed to filters that have gas residues. Some sugar-sensitive patients react to this gas and not to the sugar itself.

**PESTICIDES:** Pesticide residues are commonly found in many foods. People may tolerate unsprayed fruits but suffer severe reactions when sprayed foods are eaten. Peaches, apples, and cherries in particular are sprayed many times in a season. The pulp is so contaminated that there is no way to remove the residues. Stewing the fruit may help boil off some of the residues. Cabbage, broccoli, cauliflower, celery, lettuce, spinach, and other leafy vegetables are often heavily sprayed. To top off the contamination, fruit and vegetables may be sprayed in stores to keep off the insects and molds. Pesticide sprays also find their way into the meat supply by way of contaminated feed. Trimming fat away may reduce the contamination.

**PHENOL RESINS:** A golden brown phenol lining prevents the metal from reacting with canned foods. If you're sensitive to this, you may be able to eat some foods raw or frozen but react if they're canned.

**PLASTICS:** Commercial plastic containers and plastic wraps used by stores and homemakers may contaminate the enclosed food. Store foods and vegetables in glass containers or stainless steel. Use cellophane or parchment paper instead of plastic wraps, waxed paper, or other types. The shiny side of aluminum foil should be next to foods, not the dull side. Foil heated in ovens may release plastic fumes.

**WAXES:** A light coating of paraffin is used to make some fruits and vegetables shiny and to increase shelf life. Commonly waxed foods are parsnips, rutabagas, cucumbers, green peppers, and apples. Peeling removes some of the wax but not all

# APPENDIX D

# Carbohydrate Content of Some Common Foods

| | (in grams) |
|---|---|
| **Condiments and Dressings** | |
| Catsup (1 tablespoon) | 4.3 |
| French dressing (1 tablespoon) | 2.6 |
| Italian dressing (1 tablespoon) | 1.0 |
| Mayonnaise (1 tablespoon) | .3 |
| Mustard (1 tablespoon, prepared) | .5 |
| Relish (1 tablespoon, sweet) | 4.4 |
| Thousand Island dressing (1 tablespoon) | 2.3 |
| **Dairy Products** | |
| American cheese spread (1 ounce) | 2.3 |
| Butter (1 tablespoon) | .1 |
| Cocoa (1 cup, hot) | 27.0 |
| Cottage cheese (1 cup) | 6.5 |
| Cream (1 cup, whipping) | 7.4 |
| Egg (1 medium) | .4 |
| Ice Cream (1 cup) | 39.0 |
| Milk (1 cup, whole) | 12.0 |
| Swiss cheese (1 ounce) | .5 |
| Yogurt (1 cup, plain) | 13.0 |

| **Desserts and Sweets** | |
|---|---|
| Angel food cake (1 slice) | 24.0 |
| Apple Betty (1 serving) | 28.0 |
| Apple pie (1 piece) | 50.0 |
| Brownie with nuts (1) | 25.0 |
| Cake doughnut (1) | 17.0 |
| Caramel (1) | 3.8 |
| Chocolate chip cookie (1 medium) | 5.3 |
| Chocolate fudge (1-inch piece) | 34.0 |
| Corn syrup (1 tablespoon) | 15.0 |
| Devil's food cupcake with icing (1) | 28.0 |
| Fruit-flavored gelatin (1 cup) | 34.0 |
| Honey (1 tablespoon) | 16.0 |
| Jelly (1 tablespoon) | 14.0 |
| Jelly beans (1 ounce) | 26.0 |
| Lollipop (1 medium) | 27.0 |
| Maple syrup (1 tablespoon) | 13.0 |
| Marshmallow (1 large) | 4.7 |
| Milk chocolate bar (2 ounces) | 32.0 |
| Molasses (1 tablespoon, blackstrap) | 11.0 |
| Oatmeal cookie with raisins (1) | 14.3 |
| Pumpkin pie (1 piece) | 30.0 |
| Shortbread cookie (1 plain) | 5.4 |
| Sugar (1 tablespoon, granulated) | 12.0 |
| Vanilla pudding (1 cup) | 39.0 |
| **Fruits and Fruit Juices** | |
| Apple (1 medium, raw) | 17.0 |
| Apple cider (1 cup) | 34.4 |
| Applesauce (1 cup, unsweetened) | 23.0 |
| Banana (1 medium) | 30.0 |
| Blueberries (1 cup, canned in syrup) | 61.0 |
| Blueberries (1 cup, raw) | 19.0 |
| Cantaloupe (¼ raw) | 7.5 |
| Cranberry juice cocktail (1 cup) | 40.0 |
| Dates (1 medium) | 6.3 |
| Fruit cocktail (1 cup, canned in heavy syrup) | 47.0 |
| Grapefruit (1 medium) | 25.0 |
| Grapefruit juice (1 cup, unsweetened) | 17.0 |
| Grape juice (1 cup) | 41.0 |

| | |
|---|---|
| Grapes (1 cup, green seedless) | 27.2 |
| Lemonade (1 cup, diluted concentrate) | 27.0 |
| Lemon juice (1 tablespoon, fresh) | 1.2 |
| Nectarine (1 medium, raw) | 12.0 |
| Orange (1 medium) | 20.0 |
| Orange juice (1 cup, unsweetened) | 29.0 |
| Peach (1 medium) | 10.0 |
| Pear (1 medium) | 27.8 |
| Pineapple (1 cup, crushed, canned in syrup) | 47.0 |
| Pineapple (1 cup, raw) | 17.0 |
| Prune juice (1 cup, unsweetened) | 45.0 |
| Raisins (1 cup) | 111.0 |
| Strawberries (1 cup, raw) | 11.0 |
| Watermelon (1 cup, cubes) | 12.0 |
| **Meats, Poultry, and Seafood** | |
| Beef pot pie (4½-inch diameter) | 42.7 |
| Beef roast, steak, hamburger | 0.0 |
| Chicken, turkey, pork, or lamb (broiled or roasted) | 0.0 |
| Cod, flounder (broiled or baked) | 0.0 |
| Fishstick (1 breaded) | 1.4 |
| Scallops (4 ounces, breaded) | 12.0 |
| Tuna (in oil or water) | 0.0 |
| **Nuts and Seeds** | |
| Almonds (1 cup, dried) | 26.0 |
| Cashews (1 cup) | 26.0 |
| Peanut butter (1 tablespoon, natural) | 2.4 |
| Peanuts (1 cup, roasted) | 48.0 |
| Pecans (1 cup) | 15.2 |
| Sunflower seeds (1 cup, dried) | 19.0 |
| Walnuts (1 cup, raw) | 15.0 |
| **Oils and Fats** | |
| Margarine (1 tablespoon) | .1 |
| Vegetable oils | 0.0 |
| **Soups** | |
| Chicken noodle (1 cup) | 8.2 |
| Clam chowder (1 cup, New England) | 10.5 |

| | |
|---|---|
| Potato (1 cup, creamed) | 12.0 |
| Tomato (1 cup, creamed with milk) | 22.0 |
| Vegetable (1 cup, beef) | 9.7 |
| **Starches** | |
| Biscuits (1, 2½ inch) | 17.0 |
| Bran flakes (1 cup) | 30.8 |
| Bread (1 slice, rye or white) | 12.0 |
| Bread (1 slice, wholewheat) | 11.0 |
| Corn flakes (1 cup) | 21.0 |
| Cornmeal (1 cup, whole-ground) | 90.0 |
| Cornstarch (1 tablespoon) | 7.0 |
| Cracker (1 medium, graham) | 5.1 |
| Cracker (1, 2½ inch, soda) | 4.2 |
| Cracker (1 medium, rye) | 1.5 |
| Danish pastry (1 small) | 16.0 |
| Flour (1 cup, all-purpose) | 84.0 |
| Flour (1 cup, wholewheat) | 82.0 |
| Macaroni (1 cup, cooked) | 32.0 |
| Noodles (1 cup, cooked) | 37.0 |
| Oatmeal (1 cup, cooked) | 23.0 |
| Pizza (⅛ cheese, 14-inch diameter) | 21.0 |
| Popcorn (1 cup, popped) | 8.3 |
| Potato flour (1 cup) | 86.0 |
| Rice (1 cup, cooked, brown) | 37.0 |
| Rye flour (1 cup, medium) | 79.0 |
| Soy flour (1 cup) | 36.0 |
| Spaghetti with meat sauce (1 cup) | 38.0 |
| Wheat germ (1 tablespoon) | 2.7 |
| **Vegetables** | |
| Asparagus (1 spear, cooked) | .6 |
| Beans (1 cup, cooked, green) | 8.9 |
| Beans (1 cup, cooked, lima) | 49.0 |
| Beans (1 cup, canned, red kidney) | 42.6 |
| Broccoli (1 cup, cooked) | 6.7 |
| Cabbage (1 cup, shredded raw) | 5.7 |
| Carrot (1 large, raw) | 9.7 |
| Cauliflower (1 cup, raw) | 5.2 |
| Celery (1 large stalk, raw) | 2.0 |

| | |
|---|---|
| Corn-on-the-cob (4-inch ear) | 18.8 |
| Cucumber (½ not pared) | 1.7 |
| Lettuce (3½ ounces, iceberg) | 2.9 |
| Onion (1 raw) | .8 |
| Peas (1 cup, cooked, green) | 12.1 |
| Potato (1 medium, baked with skin) | 21.1 |
| Potato chips (1 cup) | 20.0 |
| Potatoes (1 cup, french fries) | 43.0 |
| Pumpkin (⅔ cup, canned) | 7.9 |
| Spinach (1 cup, steamed) | 3.6 |
| Sweet potato (1 small, baked) | 32.5 |
| Tomato (1 raw, medium) | 7.1 |
| Tomato juice (1 cup) | 8.6 |

All information in this appendix is based on: *Nutrition Almanac* (New York: McGraw-Hill, 1973, 1975).

# APPENDIX E

# Food Families

Here are some of the most common food families. For a more complete list, ask your librarian for a food taxonomy reference book. Don't be surprised if one book's lists differ from another's. Taxonomists do not always agree on how the animals and plants should be arranged into families.

### Animal Families

**Bird:** chicken, pheasant, quail, and their eggs; duck, goose; turkey
**Bovid:** Beef, goat, lamb, milk products
**Crustaceans:** Crab, crayfish, lobster, shrimp
**Freshwater Fish:** Bass, herring, perch, salmon, sturgeon, trout, whitefish
**Mollusks:** Abalone, clam, oyster, scallops, snail
**Saltwater Fish:** Anchovy, cod, flounder, mackerel, sea bass, sea herring, sole, tuna
**Swine:** Pork and pork products

### Plant Families

**Apple:** Apple, pear, quince
**Banana:** Arrowroot, banana, plantain
**Beet:** Beet, lamb's-quarters, spinach
**Buckwheat:** Buckwheat, rhubarb

**Cashew:** Cashew, mango, pistachio

**Citrus:** Citron, grapefruit, kumquat, lemon, lime, orange, tangerine

**Cola:** Chocolate, cocoa, cola

**Composite:** Artichoke, chicory, dandelion, endive, lettuce, sunflower

**Date:** Coconut, date

**Fungus:** Mushroom, yeast

**Ginger:** Ginger, tumeric

**Gourd:** Cantaloupe, cucumber, pumpkin, squash, watermelon, zucchini

**Grass:** Barley, cane, corn, molasses, oats, rice, rye, sorghum, wheat, wild rice

**Heather:** Blueberry, cranberry, huckleberry, wintergreen

**Laurel:** Avocado, bay leaf, cinnamon, sassafras

**Legume:** Alfalfa, bean (garbanzo [chick pea], kidney, lima, navy, pinto, string), carob, clover honey, lentil, licorice, pea (black-eyed, green), peanut, soybean, sprouts

**Lily:** Asparagus, chive, garlic, leek, onion

**Mallow:** Cottonseed, okra

**Mint:** Basil, marjoram, mint, oregano, peppermint, sage, spearmint, thyme

**Mustard:** Brussels sprouts, cabbage, cauliflower, collards, horseradish, kale, mustard, radish, rutabaga, turnip, watercress

**Myrtle:** Allspice, clove

**Nutmeg:** Nutmeg, mace

**Parsley:** Anise, caraway, carrot, celery, celery seed, coriander, cumin, dill, fennel, parsley, parsnip

**Plum:** Almond, apricot, cherry, nectarine, peach, plum, wild cherry

**Potato:** Cayenne, chili pepper, eggplant, paprika, pepper (red, green), potato, tomato

**Rose:** Blackberry, boysenberry, raspberry, strawberry

**Walnut:** Black walnut, butternut, English walnut, hickory nut, pecan

The following are food families with only one member each: Brazil nut, grape (raisin), macademia nut, maple, olive, pineapple, sesame, sweet potato, tapioca, tea, vanilla.

# APPENDIX F

# Suggested Reading

**Allergy**

Billman, Alice. *Guidelines for Ecological Living.* 1982. Available from: Human Ecology Research Foundation of the Southwest, 12110 Webbs Chapel, Suite 305E, Dallas, Tex. 75234.
(An extensive guide of well-tolerated products for the chemically susceptible person.)

Crook, William G. *Are You Allergic?* 1974. Available from: Professional Books, PO Box 3494, Jackson, Tenn. 38301.
(A super guide for the allergic person.)

———. *Tracking Down Hidden Food Allergies.* 1978. Available from: Professional Books, PO Box 3494, Jackson, Tenn. 38301.
(A well-written, well-illustrated guide, with easy-to-follow directions for detecting your food allergies.)

———. *The Yeast Connection,* 1983. Available from: Professional Books, PO Box 3494, Jackson, Tenn. 38301.
(This well-written book contains vital information and practical suggestions for overcoming yeast-related health problems.)

Dickey, Lawrence, Ed. *Clinical Ecology.* Springfield, Ill.: Charles C Thomas, 1970.

Forman, Robert. *How to Control Your Allergies.* New York: Larchmont Books, 1979.
(An excellent account of how clinical ecology can alleviate many medical conditions.)

Frazier, Claude A. *Coping with Food Allergy.* New York: Quadrangle/New York Times Book Co., 1974.
(A thorough, well-written book on food allergies, with many helpful recipes.)

Gerrard, John W. *Food Allergy: New Perspectives.* Springfield, Ill.: Charles C Thomas, 1980.
(A superb book, edited by a university professor, that presents both traditional and nontraditional views of food allergies.)

Golos, Natalie, and Golbitz, Frances. *Coping with Your Allergies.* New York: Simon & Schuster, 1978.
(A complete guide for managing complex allergies.)

———. *If This Is Tuesday It Must Be Chicken.* 1981. Available from: Human Ecology Research Foundation of the Southwest, 12110 Webbs Chapel Road, Suite 305E, Dallas, Tex. 75234.
(A must for those living on a rotation diet.)

Ludeman, Kate, and Henderson, Louise. *Do-It-Yourself Allergy Analysis Handbook.* New Canaan, Conn.: Keats Publishing, 1979.

Mackarness, Richard. *Chemical Victims.* London: Pan Books, 1980.

———. *Eating Dangerously.* New York: Harcourt Brace Jovanovich, 1976.

Mandell, Marshall, and Scanlon, Lynne. *Dr. Mandell's 5-Day Allergy Relief System.* New York: Pocket Books, 1979.
(Readers with multiple allergies will identify with the many case histories presented. Fasting is covered in detail.)

Miller, Joseph B. *Food Allergy: Provocative Testing and Injection Therapy.* Springfield, Ill.: Charles C Thomas, 1972.
(A book for physicians on the techniques of provocative testing and treatment.)

Pfeiffer, Guy O. *The Household Environment and Chronic Illness.* Springfield, Ill.: Charles C Thomas, 1980.

Philpott, William, and Kalita, Dwight K. *Brain Allergies.* New Canaan, Conn.: Keats Publishing, 1980.
(An interesting book written for both patients and their doctors.)

Randolph, Theron. *Human Ecology and Susceptibility to the Chemical Environment.* Springfield, Ill.: Charles C Thomas, 1970.
(A well-written, fascinating account by one of the pioneers in clinical ecology of how the environment can cause severe medical problems.)

Randolph, Theron and Moss, Ralph. *An Alternative Approach to Allergies.* New York: Harper & Row, 1980.
(A must for all those with chemical sensitivities.)

Rapp, Doris J. *Allergies and Your Child*. New York: Holt, Rinehart & Winston, 1972.
(A helpful book with answers to lots of questions parents of allergic children might ask.)

———. *Allergies and Your Family.* New York: Sterling Publishing, 1981.
(A complete guide in question-and-answer format for families with allergic members.)

Sheinkin, David; Schachter, Michael; and Hutton, Richard. *The Food Connection*. New York: Bobbs-Merrill, 1979.
(A well-written guide for food allergy sufferers giving alternative methods of testing and treatment.)

Truss, C. Orian. *The Missing Diagnosis.* 1983. Available from: PO Box 26508, Birmingham, Ala. 35226.
(An exciting book about the effects of chronic Candida infections by the pioneer.)

Zamm, Alfred, and Gannon, Robert. *Why Your House May Endanger Your Health.* New York: Simon & Schuster, 1980.

**Diet and Behavior**

Abrahamson, E. M., and Pezet, A. W. *Body, Mind and Sugar.* New York: Avon, 1951.

Cheraskin, E.; Ringsdorf, W. M.; and Bresher, A. *Psychodietetics.* New York: Bantam Books, 1974.

Cott, Alan. *The Orthomolecular Approach to Learning Disabilities.* 1977. Available from: Academic Therapy Publications, PO Box 899, 1539 Fourth Street, San Rafael, Cal. 94901.
(An interesting book for parents interested in diet and vitamin therapy for their learning-disabled child.)

Crook, William G. *Can Your Child Read? Is He Hyperactive?* 1975. Available from: Professional Books, PO Box 3494, Jackson, Tenn. 38301.
(A must for every parent with a hyperactive or learning-disabled child. Lots of helpful information on diet, allergy, medicines, vitamins, and behavior modification.)

Duffy, William. *Sugar Blues.* Radnor, Penna.: Chilton Book Co., 1975.

Feingold, B. F. *Why Your Child Is Hyperactive*. New York: Random House, 1974.
(An interesting book about this pioneer's work, with his additive- and salicylate-free diet for hyperactive children.)

Fredericks, Carlton, and Goodman, Herman. *Low Blood Sugar and You.* New York: Grosset & Dunlap, 1969.

New York Institute for Child Development, with Walsh, Ralph J. *Treating Your Hyperactive and Learning Disabled Child*. New York: Anchor Press, 1973.

Powers, Hugh, and Presley, James. *Food-Power: Nutrition and Your Child's Behavior.* New York: St. Martin's Press, 1978.

Rapp, Doris J. *Allergies and the Hyperactive Child*. New York: Sovereign Books, 1979.
(A well-written, helpful book for parents who have a hyperactive child.)

Schauss, Alexander, *Diet, Crime and Delinquency.* Berkeley, Cal.: Parker House, 1980.

Smith, Lendon H. *Improving Your Child's Behavior Chemistry.* Englewood Cliffs, N.J.: Prentice-Hall, 1976.
(An entertaining, fascinating book by a popular pediatrician for parents with hard-to-raise children.)

———. *Feed Your Kids Right*. New York: McGraw-Hill, 1979.
(An excellent guide for parents of hard-to-raise children who are interested in diet and vitamin therapy.)

Stevens, Laura J.; Stevens, George E.; and Stoner, Rosemary B. *How to Feed Your Hyperactive Child*. New York: Doubleday, 1977.

Stevens, Laura J., and Stoner, Rosemary B. *How to Improve Your Child's Behavior Through Diet*. New York: Doubleday, 1979.

**Diet, Nutrients, and Health**

Blanchard, Edward B., and Epstein, Leonard H. A. *Biofeedback Primer.* Reading, Mass: Addison-Wesley, 1978.

Brown, Barbara B. *New Mind, New Body.* New York: Harper & Row, 1974.

Coffin, Lewis, *The Grandmother Conspiracy Exposed*. Santa Barbara, Cal.: Capra Press, 1974.

(A thought-provoking book by a pediatrician who is concerned about the effect of diet on the health of today's children.)

Davis, Adelle. *Let's Have Healthy Children.* New York: Harcourt Brace Jovanovich, 1951.

Goldbeck, Nikki, and Goldbeck, David. *The Supermarket Handbook: Access to Whole Foods.* New York: Harper & Row, 1973.

Graedon, Joe. *The People's Pharmacy.* New York: Avon, 1976.
(An excellent guide to prescription and over-the-counter drugs.)

———. *The People's Pharmacy*-2. New York: Avon, 1980.
(An interesting, helpful sequel to the author's first book.)

Huggins, Hal A. *How to Balance the Chemistry of the Periodontal Patient.* 1981. Available from: HAH Publications, Box 2589, Colorado Springs, Colo. 80906.

———. *Why Raise Ugly Kids?* Westport, Conn.: Arlington House, 1981.
(Some interesting, revolutionary ideas about raising children by one of the pioneer dentists interested in balancing body chemistry.)

Hunter, Beatrice Trum. *Fact/Book on Food Additives and Your Health.* New Canaan, Conn.: Keats Publishing, 1972.

Jacobson, Michael F. *Eater's Digest: The Consumer's Factbook of Food Additives.* Garden City, N.Y.: Doubleday Anchor Books, 1972.

———. *Nutrition Scoreboard.* New York: Avon Books, 1974.

Lesser, Michael. *Nutrition and Vitamin Therapy.* New York: Grove Press, 1980.
(One of the best books available on vitamin and mineral therapy for those with mental symptoms.)

Mindell, Earl. *Vitamin Bible.* New York: Warner Books, 1979.

Newbold, H. L. *Mega-Nutrients for Your Nerves.* New York: Wyden, 1978.

Nutrition Search. *Nutrition Almanac.* New York: McGraw-Hill, 1975.

Oski, Frank. *Don't Drink Your Milk.* New York: Wyden, 1977.

Ott, John H. *Health and Light.* Old Greenwich, Conn.: Devin-Adair Co., 1973.
(A fascinating account of the effects of light on animals and plants and how modern lighting, building, and television may affect our health adversely.)

Passwater, Richard A. *Evening Primrose Oil.* New Canaan, Conn.: Keats Publishing, 1981.

Pfeiffer, Carl C. *Mental and Elemental Nutrients.* New Canaan, Conn.: Keats Publishing, 1975.

Reader's Digest. *Eat Better, Live Better.* Pleasantville, N.Y.: Reader's Digest Association, 1982.

Schroeder, Henry A. *The Poisons Around Us.* Bloomington: Indiana University Press, 1974.
(An excellent reference book about toxic metals.)

Smith, Lendon H. *Foods for Healthy Kids.* New York: McGraw-Hill, 1981.
(An excellent guide for parents interested in good nutrition for their children.)

William, Roger J. *Nutrition Against Disease.* New York: Pitman Publishing, 1971.

———, and Kalita, Dwight K. *A Physician's Handbook on Orthomolecular Medicine.* Elmsford, N.Y.: Pergamon, 1977.

Wright, Jonathan V. *Dr. Wright's Book of Nutritional Therapy.* Emmaus, Penna.: Rodale Press, 1979.
(An informative book by a doctor who uses nutritional remedies in his practice whenever possible.)

# RECIPE INDEX

# SUBJECT INDEX